ONE HUNDRED
DOSES

ONE HUNDRED DOSES

Capsules of Advice and Wisdom
for the Health and Well-being
of Farm and Ranch Women

Teddy Jones and Sue Jane Sullivan

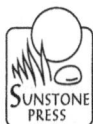

SUNSTONE
PRESS

SANTA FE

Sunstone books may be purchased for educational, business, or sales
promotional use. For information please write: Special Markets Department,
Sunstone Press, P.O. Box 2321, Santa Fe, New Mexico 87501-2321.

Library of Congress Cataloging -in-Publication Data

Jones, Teddy, 1943-
    One hundred doses : capsules of advice and wisdom for the health
and well-being of farm and ranch women / by Teddy Jones and Sue Jane
Sullivan.
        p. cm.
    ISBN 0-86534-460-4 (softcover : alk. paper)
    1. Women farmers—Health and hygiene—United States. 2. Women
ranchers—Health and hygiene—United States. 3. Rural women—Health
and hygiene—United States. 4. Self-care, Health. I. Sullivan, Sue Jane.
II. Title.

RA778.J626 2005
613'.04244—dc22

                                                    2005017612

Published in

WWW.SUNSTONEPRESS.COM
SUNSTONE PRESS / POST OFFICE BOX 2321 / SANTA FE, NM 87504-2321 /USA
(505) 988-4418 / ORDERS ONLY (800) 243-5644 / FAX (505) 988-1025

The authors gratefully acknowledge the use
of brief excerpts from the following:

Griffith, Nanci and R. West (1994) "Trouble in the Fields"
copyright Irving Music/Wing and Wheel Music from
"The MCA Years: A Retrospective" copyright 1994 MCA
(Used with permission)

Williams, Margery (1975) *The Velveteen Rabbit* New York:
Avon Books, p. 16,17 (Used with permission)

Contents

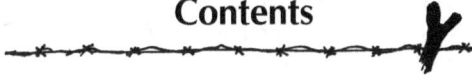

III / Take As Needed

"Take As Needed" recognizes that the unexpected occurs. Essays in this section offer advice for dealing with those out-of-the-ordinary challenges. The variety of topics emphasizes actions that can protect and improve your health and help you understand potential threats to your well-being.

IV / Give Frequently To Family And Friends

The needs of others' health and well-being are part of your scope of influence. Read the articles in "Give Frequently To Family and Friends" for support in guiding those important to you toward their best.

V / Apply Liberally To Your Community

This final section reminds that although you may live ten minutes from your nearest neighbor and half an hour from the grocery store, you are part of a community. Regardless of physical distances between and among us, our lives are interrelated. Improving any of us improves all of us. The community depends on you and can benefit from your efforts to assure its health. These essays emphasize the value of community and suggest methods to bolster its well-being.

Acknowledgments

*M*any people provided material for this book. Some did so intentionally by sharing stories of their lives and of their families. Others were unaware of their importance as sources of ideas or inspiration, primarily because I caught them being themselves and let their concerns, questions, and humor suggest topics for advice on promoting health. Thank you to each one.

Thanks also to J.T. Smith and Dan Crummett of *The Farmer Stockman*. They have welcomed the columns I have written for the pages of that magazine. Many of my pieces in this book have appeared in a slightly different form in that column, "In the Middle Of It All."

My co-author has been a delight to work with. Collaboration has seldom been so pleasant for me as has this endeavor. Thank you—Sue Jane.

And thanks to my husband Jim Bob Jones for making it possible for me to be a farm/ranch woman and for encouraging me to be and do whatever I am capable of.

—Teddy Jones

*T*o my Wednesday night church ladies. Staying in touch with you led to this writing project.

To Borden County. Teaching your children has been the great joy of my life.

To Mom and Dad. Being loved and nurtured by you gave me the security that all children should have.

To Scotty, Sara, Shane, and Sabrina, my brothers and sisters. Laughing with you, and at you, has made our family's dysfunctional moments bearable.

To Teddy. Holding your writer's hand the past few months has given me confidence and a new friend.

To Julie and Emily. Being Mom to you just makes it all complete.

—Sue Jane Sullivan

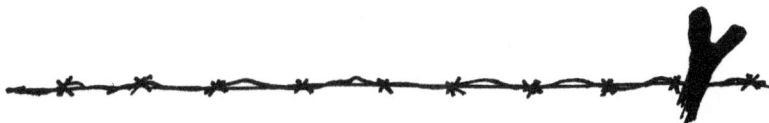

Introduction

A farm or ranch woman's day is often long and frequently demanding. There's none of the predictable routine of an administrative job, although you may be the administrator who keeps the books for your operation; there's no scheduled "free period" like the school teacher's designated time to grade papers and plan lessons although you may home-school your children; five o'clock doesn't necessarily signal the end of your "shift"; and your work day often begins long before salespeople report for work in retail stores. But the long hours and the enormity of the scope of your work can be more than balanced by the benefits of a life close to the land. On the tough days you can remind yourself of harvest, of roundup, of shearing, of shipping, of the beauty of the ever-changing cycles of nature, and of the satisfactions of seeing directly the effects of your effort.

Even though your days may be somewhat unpredictable, there are some recurring elements, things that are repeated almost every day. Depending on the organization of your agricultural life and your family's needs, those constant elements may include child care, animal care, and most important of all, must include self-care.

You can meet the demands of your busy life, your important role in your family and community, only if you take good care of yourself—body, mind, and spirit. The purpose of this book is to encourage you, perhaps to make you smile, and to provide useful information about caring for yourself. In the same fashion that medications or supplements are used; some daily, some less frequently; the essays in this book are grouped according to the frequency with which their content might be needed. There is no plot, but rather this is a collection of brief pieces that address topics important to the health and well-being of farm and ranch women and that do so from the perspectives of two of your "sisters."

According to the 2002 Census of Agriculture, 847, 680 women in the United States are considered operators of farms. Of those, 62% are identified

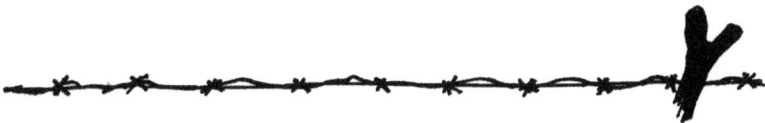

as second or third operators of the farm, suggesting that they are part of a family farm operation. There are no equivalent data for the ranching industry, but most ranches are considered farms for the purpose of this census, in which "farm" is defined as agricultural land used for crops, pasture, or grazing. Beyond those listed in this current census, there are a vast number of women who grew up on farms or ranches who may live elsewhere but continue to think of themselves as from this heritage. Other women who relate strongly to the lives of farm and ranch women are those who live and work in the small rural towns that are the community focus for farm and ranch people. Their lives are intertwined with the farmers' and ranchers' by virtue of being the teachers, health care personnel, merchants and service providers in rural towns.

This book is for and about all of you—its capsules are good for the health and well-being of every farm or ranch woman.

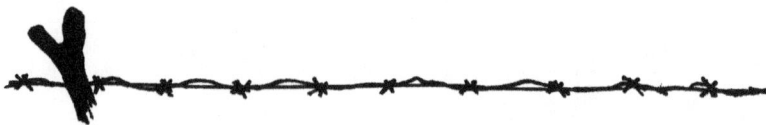

Capsule 1

Ease Into The Day

*L*et's peek over her shoulder. She won't notice because she's getting organized. The day's "to do" list she's writing shows that her life is a lot like yours or mine. A farm or ranch woman can find plenty of variety if she wants it. Regardless of whether she's a solo operator or a partner/spouse; whether she attends primarily to indoor or outdoor work or some of everything, there's always plenty for that list.

It looks like the woman we're spying on is part of a two-person operation and one who can be found working both outdoors and inside, depending on the time of day and season of the year. Ah, she's very organized—her list has time estimates for each chore. So far the list includes:

1. Untarp and climb into grain cart to clean out sprouts in preparation for loading seed wheat—1 hour
2. Baby sit 18 month-old Jason Carey this p.m.—1 hour
3. Drive tractor to shred weeds on CRP acres—3 hours
4. Take dogs for daily two-mile walk/run. Work on training on sit and stay—45 minutes
5. Input data for records and accounts—30 minutes
6. Write article for newsletter; put on disk—1.5 hours
7. Cook supper—30 minutes
8. Laundry

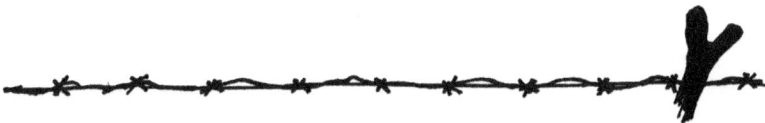

9. Go to town for mail; pick up seed lubricant—45 minutes
10. Check on sick calf 3 times—1 hour

Let's leave her alone. She's got work to do. I hope she doesn't think of another hour-long chore for that list. If she asked me, I would have a suggestion, though. I'd encourage her to add just one other thing that might make the more-than-ten-hour day she's outlined less of a strain. "Ease into it," I'd say. "Take some time to stretch before you begin to run, walk, climb, lift, stoop, drive, and bend."

Before you object on her behalf, saying she doesn't have time for one more thing, let me explain.

Stretching all the major muscle groups is a gentle, relaxing way to maintain and improve flexibility and balance. A flexible body is less prone to injury from the movement performed in the variety of work we do. The list we peeked at included both indoor and outdoor activities. Everything from climbing into the grain bin, lifting a child, carrying the laundry, bending to get pots from the cabinet, to working seated at the computer and driving the tractor requires flexibility. No muscle group was exempt from work and no joint went unused. Stretching does not produce strength or endurance, but it does help make motion more fluid and reduces risk of injury. Posture improves and gravity loses some of its attraction. That woman should stretch! In fact, each of us should, every day or at least three times a week.

You notice the woman we were observing is younger than you? No matter. Any age is a good age to begin stretching. You'll notice that young athletes are taught to do it. For that matter, young animals do it without any instruction. If you've not been a stretcher, you'll find that developing flexibility takes some time. Be gentle with yourself and expect that improvement will be gradual. In a few days time you'll see progress and in a few weeks you'll be amazed by the change. If age or injuries, chronic illness, or joint replacements have altered your mobility, check

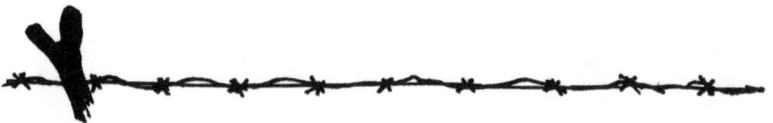

with your health care provider about any special precautions before you begin stretching.

There's no perfect stretching routine. Yoga and Tai Chi are formal methods that incorporate all the benefits of stretching. But you can also develop your own way. Be certain to include the following principles:

- ✪ The routine can be performed lying, sitting, standing, or in some combination of those.
- ✪ Begin stretching only after walking around and swinging your arms to increase blood flow—warm up a little.
- ✪ Hold each stretch 15 to 20 seconds and repeat each position three times.
- ✪ Do not bounce or twist violently.
- ✪ If any movement causes more than a pulling sensation, reduce the stretch. Proper stretching should not produce pain.
- ✪ Start at the top with head and neck and work down. Each movement should be paralleled by the same movement on the opposite side of the body.
- ✪ Stretch the neck through all its positions—look up, down, and over each shoulder.
- ✪ Shrug the shoulders and arch the back.
- ✪ Lift the arms high, reaching above the head. Next bend one elbow and grasp it with the opposite hand. Pull behind the head toward the grasping hand until stretching is felt in the upper arm, shoulder and down the side. Continue the gentle pull while leaning sideways from the waist toward the grasping hand. Now that's a stretch.
- ✪ Face forward and twist gently to rotate the trunk to one side. Open the arms at shoulder level. As you rotate, keep the arm on the side you are turning to open and cross the other over the chest toward the open arm. You should be looking behind you by now!

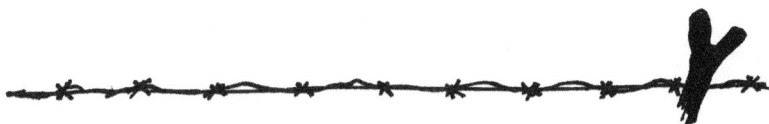

- Elongate the vertical back muscles by bending forward at the hips.
- Cross a leg over the other one to pull on the hip muscles (lying or standing).
- Stretch hamstring muscles at the back of the thigh by lifting the leg nearly perpendicular at the hip with the knee almost straight. Keep the back straight also. It's not cheating to use the hands to lift the leg.
- Quadriceps, muscles at the front of the thigh, are worked by bending the knee and grasping the ankle behind you. Hold on to a chair back for balance if needed.
- Calf muscles and heel tendons are lengthened by lifting the toes toward the head. If standing, raise the foot forward off the floor about four inches. Opposing muscles are worked in the same position by lifting the heel toward the calf and pointing the toes.

As you master the basics, add some other positions just for fun. Pretend you're a dancer. Use the top of the kitchen cabinet or a fence rail at about waist height as a "barre" to put your foot on. Facing your "barre" try to put your head to your knee on the raised leg by reaching, ever so gracefully, for your foot. Or reach for the top of a doorway and stand on tiptoes. You get the point—to work every muscle and joint gently and to feel the stretch.

The benefits of stretching don't depend on the time of day—anytime is good. Some people manage to fit stretching into their day by taking advantage of small breaks in their activities; five minutes here, ten minutes there. But if you can avoid hitting the floor running each morning, twenty minutes devoted to stretching is a beneficial, quiet way to start the day. It's a way to just ease into it.

—Teddy

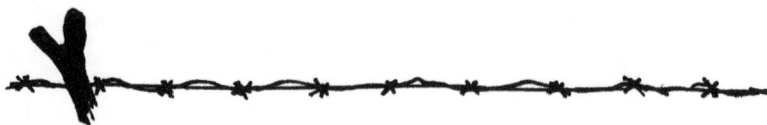

Capsule 2

Just Walk Away

*T*hose words, "Just walk away," contain some pithy advice: how to avoid an argument you can't win; how to avoid temptation; what to do when your tractor seizes up and grinds to a halt and the sledge hammer won't cure it; when if you didn't have bad luck, you wouldn't have any luck at all; when your last emu goes down with some rare avian disease. It is multipurpose wisdom, useful in so many situations. Taken just slightly differently, "Just walk a *way,*" the phrase also encourages a simple and highly effective health promoting action.

Walking is one of the very best forms of exercise a person can get. No need to run, just put one foot in front of the other and head out. Research shows that you can improve your blood pressure, your muscle tone, your heart and lung function and your stress level by walking. And walking helps keep your weight right, too. Digestion improves as does bowel function. Walking gets the blood coursing around the circulatory system, burns calories, and can help a person with diabetes keep their glucose level in desired range.

Do all of those benefits sound like the "too good to be true" sort of claims made for some patent medicines? What's the catch? As far as I can see, there's only one. Walking takes more time than taking a pill. But, maybe it doesn't take as much time as you might think. Researchers say that walking just 20-30 minutes three times a week has significant

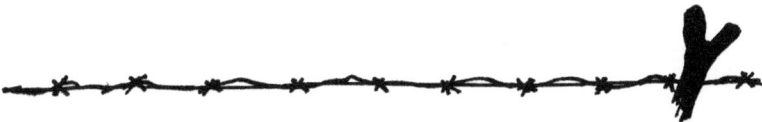

benefits. Increase that time and/or increase to five days and you increase the benefits. Don't worry about the distance. Aim for time and for increasing your speed as days go by.

There are some choices you can make that will encourage you to get in the habit of walking more in general, in addition to your "planned walks." For example, you can park in the farthest row from the door when you go to public places such as the grocery store or to church. If someone in your family is eligible for the disabled parking sticker on your car or pickup, resist the urge to always pull into the handy blue striped space in front of the door. If you are not the disabled person, don't use the parking space.

When a person first starts walking farther than the mailbox, some caution is in order. Stretch your muscles a little each time before you start, to prevent soreness. Wear good athletic shoes that are comfortable and some nice padded socks that wick up perspiration.

If you don't want to go alone and you find that no one else is as health-conscious as you are, take your pet. Well, I guess that depends on what kind of pet you have. Getting a cat to walk is a little tough, but most dogs will love it. Or you can take a portable radio or tape player and have any kind of company you want. I'm fond of Delbert McClinton and ZZ Top. Maybe you would prefer Bob Wills.

Walk where? That all depends on your mood. You can go around the same two-block stretch several times. (Good manners *do not* require you to say hi to the neighbor who is looking out her window each time you make the block.) Or, you can choose a new route to explore each time. Some people go to the mall to walk, but I think it is very tempting to dawdle in the mall. Besides, the only thing mall-like in lots of our rural towns is the grocery store-gas station complex near the only traffic light. Other people invest in a treadmill. That's nice when the weather is bad. No excuse then. And of course there is always the nearest county road. Don't forget that trucks hauling manure or ensilage have the right of way.

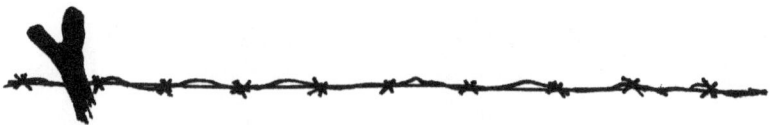

Some people feel that having arthritis prevents them from walking. If the arthritis affects knees or hips, then care must be taken not to walk so far or so fast as to overtire the joint and its surrounding muscles, ligaments and tendons. If the joint is currently inflamed and swollen, it should be rested and some other form of exercise would be better. But, if a person observes the "stretch before you walk" rule and wears good supportive shoes with a cushioned sole, the walk can actually increase circulation and improve function by reducing stiffness.

When you get back from that walk there are a couple of important things to do. First, refresh yourself with a big glass of water. You need to replace fluid used by the exercise. Second, congratulate yourself. You have just done something that is really good for your health.

So what's stopping you? If you're like most of us, it's just one step: the first step out the door. Go ahead and take that step. Just walk away.

—Teddy

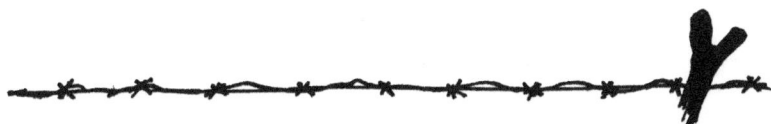

Capsule 3

Walking and Prayer

*I*n my mundane but basically peaceful world in Borden County, every now and then I walk on the track at the football field. The other day, while pacing myself in lane 7, it occurred to me that perhaps I had ADD (attention deficit disorder) when it came to praying. My mind, even in the best of serene circumstances, just bounces from thought to thought. Prozac can only do so much. This is frustrating because I want to talk to God, like to talk to God, and do talk to God, but bless His heart, even God has to have difficulty following my train of prayer thought.

I have devised a plan—and now share this with you absolutely free of charge—for walking and praying at the same time.

I decided that lap number one is to be devoted to thanksgiving. The first 400 yards will be solely for the purpose of praise and thanksgiving for the blessings in my life. Lap two will be the request lap—prayers of physical healing for some, security for others, comfort for those hurting, and the usual plea for rain. Lap three is for forgiveness. I started to make it the last lap, but if I did that, I would be walking all night long, and who wants to weigh 120 pounds anyway? I often find my pace slows some in this lap as I confess and recall those things that I struggle with— chronic faults or the daily ones. This lap addresses those shortcomings.

Finally, lap four is my conversational split—my favorite, because

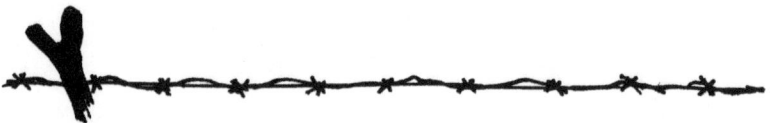

it's when God and I really visit. I tell Him what I think and feel to the core. Sometimes I think of funny things to tell Him just so He can smile; other times I just look up and marvel at the beautiful evening sky—which is like saying, "Good job." Even God needs a compliment now and then.

Tongue-in-cheek? Maybe. Look closely, though, and you'll see the Lord's Prayer outlined somewhere in there. Honor. Thanksgiving. Petitions. Forgivenness. Topped off with what's equivalent to a child jumping up into his or her parent's lap for a pre-bedtime conversation.

Whether I am walking around a track or lying in bed or driving down the road, it is an humbling realization to know that prayer is something I can do that Jesus did. And even if I lose my train of thought or fall asleep while talking to God, it's okay. Prayer, like walking a mile, is good for my heart.

—Sue Jane

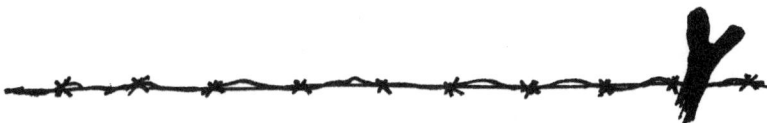

Capsule 4

Let Me Make This Perfectly Clear

*W*hen someone says "Let me make this perfectly clear," particularly if it is a politician, I expect to be confused very soon. I remember explanations "to make it perfectly clear," for new taxes, for changes in the Farm Program, and for reasons for fluctuations in the commodity markets, to mention only a few. Not a one of those left me anywhere near "clear" in my understanding. Even so, that phrase seems to me to be a very useful one to recall. Let me tell you about it and see if you might also find it worth remembering.

There are few of us who did not learn in health class that we should drink six to eight glasses of water every day. But there are lots of us who never approach that amount of water or of any other fluid each day. Maybe that is true for a number of reasons. Water that tastes bad isn't likely to attract me. Convenience is another problem, particularly if your farm and ranch work keeps you in the field all day. If it's not there, we don't drink it. Some people drink only when they feel thirsty, so if it isn't hot, they may not notice thirst. And then there is the problem of having to urinate more often if we drink more fluid. Busy people just hate to stop, for anything.

There are some good reasons why a person should drink adequate fluids (and why we heard that in health class and on nightly news medical updates). First, every cell in the body has to have water to transport

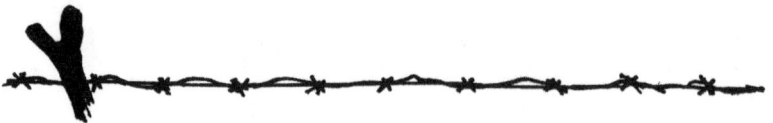

nutrients to it and to carry waste products away. Without sufficient fluid, cells function more slowly and wastes collect. So, a person who is dehydrated is poorly coordinated, thinks more slowly, and risks reduced blood volume. Reduced blood volume means that organs do not receive adequate nutrients and oxygen for their function. That means every organ. The bowels reduce function, so digestion is poor and constipation occurs. Heart, lungs and kidneys try to compensate for the volume problems and the reduced nutrients and oxygen and, as a result, are placed under the strain of overwork. The skin is affected too. A person chronically low on fluids has dry skin that wrinkles more easily and heals more slowly. If someone tried to damage us in these ways, by giving us a poison, we would all resist very actively!

But wait, there are other problems that go along with reduced fluid intake. People who have a history of kidney stones or of urinary tract infections are taking a big chance of recurrences of those problems if they limit their fluids. And a person with gout needs lots of fluids to reduce those painful joint problems.

Does it have to be water? The first concern is adequate fluid for the body to extract water. So, plain water is the easiest way to get that. But, sports drinks, fruit juices, milk and other non-caffeinated fluids can count in the daily intake total. The key point is that the fluid is non-caffeinated. Since caffeine has a diuretic effect, it takes fluid out at a rate greater than it replaces it. Alcohol has a similar effect. So, if a person drinks caffeine or alcohol, they should remember to make up that loss by drinking the same amount of water. Yes, every beer means a glass of water.

It seems simple just to decide to drink more water or other fluids, but we all know that any change in habits is hard to stick to. So, a bit of thinking about why we don't get enough fluid can help a person succeed. For example, if you just don't like the taste of what your municipal water supply produces, you can get a filter pitcher that takes out some of the

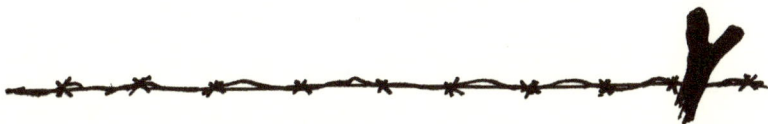

minerals that cause the taste. Or, you can buy bottled water from the machines in many grocery stores for about 25 cents a gallon. Or, if you prefer that "designer water," you can pay lots more for some cute little bottles.

If convenience is the main problem for you, then you should get at least one good container that you can carry with you every day. A quart size canteen fits into a small cooler or a good thermos type bottle keeps your drink at a tasty temperature. You can also try to get into the habit of drinking one of those daily glasses at each meal. But, carrying water along is very important if you spend your day in the field or in and out of the pickup.

Waiting for thirst to prompt taking a drink is a habit to break. Even in cold weather, a person loses fluid, not only in urine, but also in every breath exhaled. If a person waits until their tongue is dry enough to make them feel thirsty, they are dangerously low on fluid. And I can only say, "Get over it," to the person who says, "I'm just too busy to stop for a bathroom break, so I don't like to drink much." A bathroom break is also an opportunity to stretch the muscles, to change our focus (relax a bit), and to enjoy the fact that you are where you are.

You may be wondering about now just what all of that had to do with "making it perfectly clear." Well, here it is. That phrase—make it perfectly clear—is a way to be sure that you are getting enough fluid. Six to eight glasses (that is about two quarts) is enough for most people under usual circumstances, although more is better. But, heavy exercise, high intake of caffeine or alcohol, and outdoor activity in extreme weather can all increase fluid needs. The way to make certain you have enough? Check your urine—"make it perfectly clear," at least once a day.

—Teddy

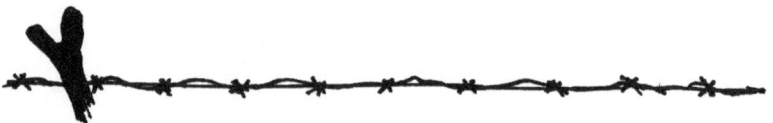

Capsule 5

Eight Glasses

We learn at a young age that drinking eight glasses of water a day is good for us. Consuming water is recommended by doctors, coaches, and personal trainers (we all have one of those, don't we?)

I fail miserably in this area. I know it's good for my body, but I'd rather drink a diet soft drink. It is self-indulgence and a lack of discipline, pure and simple. I drink carbonated beverages when I should be drinking water.

Until I get really thirsty.

It may be on a hot summer evening after mowing the yard, or from a dry mouth caused by some medicine, or a result of a bite into something spicy. At those times, nothing but water quenches my thirst.

I wish I could say that my spiritual and mental thirst were different, but I'm afraid the parallel is obvious.

The Catch 22 for today's farm and ranch woman is that modern technology has enabled her to have more free time than women 50 years ago. The chores remain much the same, but there is a machine now to do the milking, a machine to do the laundry, a microwave to help with the cooking, and computer programs to do the books.

So, with the physical demands eased somewhat, women are left with more time to devote to their spiritual and mental needs, right?

Too many times I just take sips. Whether it's a quick prayer or a

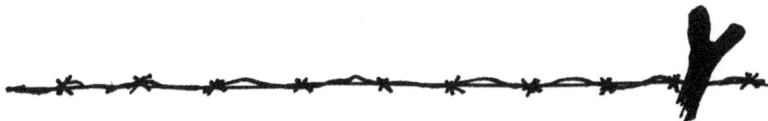

short nap or a phone visit with a friend, I find myself not having time so I simply do what little I can. The thirst isn't there, so I don't drink.

But I know that a key to health is to "drink" even when we aren't thirsty.

Our lives may have comfortable moments with few problems. Drink anyway.

We may have overcome some difficulty and seen a crisis pass. Drink anyway.

Then, when the parched times come and the real thirst returns—and it will–that living stream will be there from which to drink. Nothing will taste sweeter.

"As the deer pants for streams of water, so my soul pants for you, O God." Psalm 42:1

A woman's physical and spiritual needs are often intertwined. The routine of taking care of both areas will go a long way to easing the many demands that come with living and working on a farm or ranch.

Raise your glasses and lift your spirits.

—Sue Jane

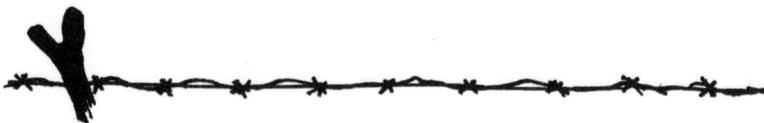

Capsule 6

Straight Ahead

"When you come to a place where you have to
go left or right," says Sister Ruth, "go straight ahead."
Dakota, Kathleen Norris

*T*he last two times I have been to Mexico, I drove my own car.
It really is no different from driving in Lubbock, Texas. So, I just imagine
myself on that city's chronic road construction, and it's "no problema."

My command of the Spanish language is not fluent, but I can
hold my own. Even people with a small grasp of the language usually
know that *derecha* means "right" and *izquierda* means "left"—two very
important words to know when taking instructions from backseat Spanish-
speaking passengers.

Driving my little Honda Civic, weaving in and out of traffic, I
was feeling pretty darn sassy on the first of these trips south to Chihuahua.
I heard *derecho* and confidently, and smugly, began to move right one
lane over.

My passenger repeated the instruction, so I changed lanes once
again to the right. I became somewhat concerned after the third utterance
of this command because there were no more right lanes. The street
vendors did not need me on their curbs to help with sales.

"No, Ud. no sabe, señora." (I'll say I didn't know.) "*Derecho* es

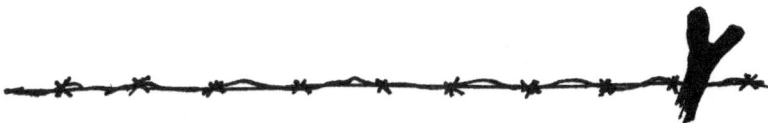

'straight ahead!'" One little letter at the end of the word—*derecho*, not *derecha*—had changed the meaning.

There have been times when I have ignored a voice that said, "Go straight ahead." I wandered, not wanting to ask for instructions, searching for what I knew to be the way to go. Surely changing one little thing from life's little book of instructions would not matter. Sometimes I even have had the arrogance to think I had no changes to make at all.

The little things, however, do matter. Mistakes and their consequences should teach us that. It is no wonder that the peace as we know it comes along a "straight and narrow" path. Straight and narrow does not mean it is difficult to get on; it just means it's a challenge to stay on—sort of like a balance beam.

That may be why we need to swallow pride and let someone hold our hand—or sit in the front seat and tell us where to go.

—Sue Jane

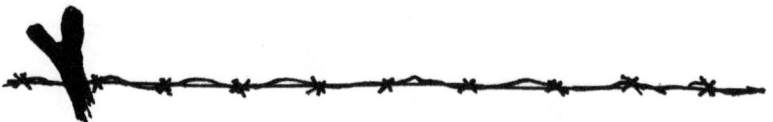

Capsule 7

The Parable of the Ol' Mutt

The small farming community in Fisher County was not my destination on this crisp October morning, but I had to pass through to get to where I was headed. Small towns like Rotan, Texas, are well past their primes, but the communities survive. The biggest draw for social activity remains the school, and it was a school activity that had brought me here on a Saturday.

Only dogs and elderly people are out and about early on a weekend in Rotan. Sure enough, I saw both near the Allsup's, the local convenience store, as they were preparing to cross the highway.

Since small towns don't need crosswalks (it's just understood that cars are to defer to the pedestrian), I slowed and stopped for both. Each had a limp, but the man's gait was characteristic of his age; the dog appeared to have a temporary sticker-in-the-paw affliction.

I felt sorry for the dog but drove on, quite content to enjoy some time to myself with my music on this peaceful morning of back road driving. But even Johnny Cash's latest CD couldn't drown out the pity, tenderheartedness and guilt. So, I decided to u-turn, see if I could locate the poor animal, save the day, and then continue with my trip.

I headed straight back to the Allsup's, but there was no sign of the wounded. No glimpse either on the neighborhood streets as I drove

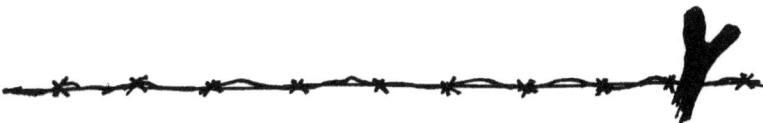

slowly around the block in search of the animal, a good deed and mostly peace of mind.

After a few minutes, I realized how suspicious I probably looked—a strange car in a small town, driving at a snail's pace, looking in people's yards and alleys. It was time to get out of Dodge and back on the farm-to-market road and risk feeling guilty rather than being arrested.

With one last glance in the Allsup's parking lot, I spotted the dog between two parked pickups. The limp was gone. Whatever had been hurting him had been removed. Someone else, or perhaps even the dog himself, had removed the hurt.

Small town living affords many such opportunities because everyone knows everyone, even their dogs. People often need help and they get it, without even having to ask. It isn't about saving the world, but just doing what comes naturally. There are sticker-pullin' moments all around us wherever we live—a simple concept that could do wonders in a complex world.

—Sue Jane

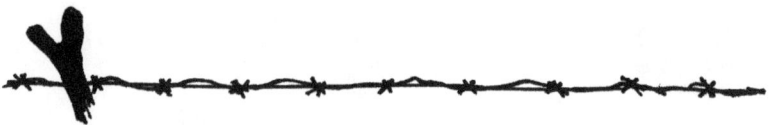

Capsule 8

Cranky No More

Our first mission the other morning at eight was to go to the implement dealership to pick up our elderly combine. The essential parts were working fine, but the air conditioner wasn't. What with the wheat looking pretty pitiful, Mr. Jones thought that baking in the cab was likely to make him a little cranky. So, the folks at the implement house had restored the "indoor air quality." A few minutes after he went inside, my husband returned smiling, carrying a bag of fresh popcorn! "Popcorn for breakfast," I said. It set me thinking. "I'll bet there's not a cranky guy in there." Why? Simple. They're eating breakfast. I will admit that popcorn's not a traditional meal, but it could go a long way toward reducing morning problems (including crankiness) caused by not eating breakfast.

Here's the way it works. Overnight, the body uses, in its own quiet way, most of the readily available glucose from your last meal. After the simple sugars (chocolate pie, for example) are used, then your liver sets to work converting the products of digested complex carbohydrates to glucose. Those are used next. (That would be the baked potato and whole wheat roll.) Next used are the protein and fats. Generally, those are stored (I can look behind me and see part of the storage!) for later conversion to glucose, if needed. All this is going on all the time, and it is obviously a lot more complicated than I am making it seem. But, the point is that the food we is eventually converted to

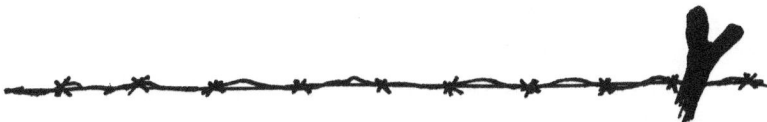

glucose for fuel and that fuel is being used all the time to operate all our functions, including the brain.

The human body is more intricate than our old combine, but they are both very sturdy and can both tolerate some bad conditions. But, the body will not tolerate a low fuel situation very well. Low blood glucose is the result when we have not eaten frequently enough or are choosing a poor combination of food. It is *normal* for the blood glucose (blood sugar) to drop when the available and stored glucose run low. One such time is after being without food overnight. One result of this low fuel situation is difficulty concentrating; a feeling of fatigue, maybe even shakiness; a problem with coordination; *and crankiness.*

A factor that compounds some of those "low blood sugar" aggravations, including crankiness, is insulin. The body requires insulin to make use of glucose at each cell. So, in a person with normal insulin function (not having diabetes), a certain amount of insulin is produced to match the amount of "floating glucose." But, for some reason coffee and other caffeine-containing items stimulate the body to push out extra insulin. The result is that if a person drinks coffee all morning and eats little or nothing, there's nothing there for the insulin to work with. They get an exaggeration of those low blood glucose signs—shaky, cranky, etc.!

A good breakfast would include a little quick simple glucose and some complex carbohydrate, a bit of protein would be good, but not absolutely essential. If you attend to those fuel requirements, you can also get some vitamins and fiber at the same time.

Simple sugar (glucose) is found in fruit juice, fruit, table sugar, jelly, and syrup, among other things. Complex carbohydrates include whole grain items like cereal, bread, bagel, muffins, breakfast bars, *and popcorn.* Some sources of protein are milk, cheese, meat, and eggs. So, there are lots of foods to choose from.

I 'm not asking you to give up anything, as lots of health promotion

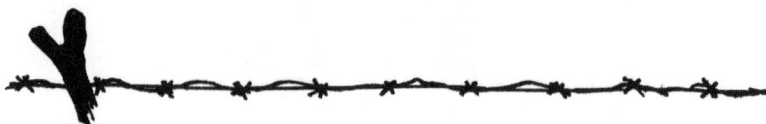

advice does. Instead, I ask you to think about what discourages you from choosing healthy actions and then to find a way to make it easier to make the positive choices. Today's challenge is how to make eating something for breakfast seem easy. Typical reasons people give for not eating breakfast are:

- I don't want to cook or don't have time.
- I'm not hungry when I wake up.

Good reasons. Let's deal with the "I'm not hungry" issue. Just pick up one or two items from each of the first two groups (simple sugars and complex carbohydrates). Remember to go heaviest on the complex carbs, because they are broken down more slowly and last longer.

A banana and a bagel would do. A box of raisins, a piece of cheese and a couple of crackers would also give you a start. You can eat those one at a time over a period of a couple of hours. It will keep your fuel level up.

As for the "I don't have time and I don't want to cook" reason, I have the perfect answer. Put an orange in your pocket and go over to the implement dealership. They're serving popcorn for breakfast. And there's not a cranky person in sight.

—Teddy

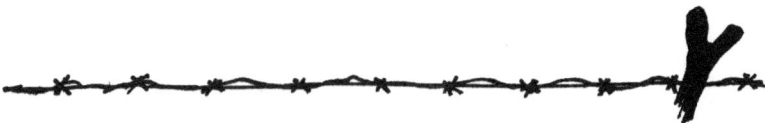

Capsule 9

Getting More Grain

*I*f that title suggests that this article will help you increase your farm's yield for wheat, corn or rice, then I'm glad it got your attention. But, to be honest, I don't have that information. If I did, then we could guarantee 100-bushel wheat this year here at Jones Farm. I hope you will read on, though, because what I do have is facts about why grains are important to our health.

You are probably aware that the nutrition information that many of us learned as youngsters has been vastly improved by research. Gone are the "Four Basic Food Groups" of our youth, replaced by the "Food Guide Pyramid." This pyramid is the method used to explain the recommended food intake requirements for all of us over the age of two years. The Pyramid accompanies the "Dietary Guidelines for Americans" issued every five years by the federal government. The most recent revision is the 2005 version.

Back to the Pyramid. Imagine one—broad base, pointy top. When I mention grains, it's the entire base of the pyramid, what all the rest is built on, that I am speaking of. Some other time we can look at the other five segments of the pyramid in more detail. Those parts are fruits; vegetables; milk, yogurt, and cheese; meat, poultry, fish, eggs, dry beans and nuts; and fats, oils, and sweets. They all are important as parts of a balanced diet. The pyramid was chosen because the number of

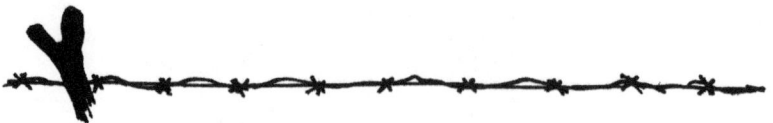

recommended servings for each group stack neatly atop one another to resemble its shape. And there's grain (bread, cereal, rice and pasta) at the base, with four to eleven recommended servings each day. The number of suggested servings varies from the lower number (four) for a 1200 calorie daily intake to the higher (eleven) for a 2800 calorie diet. The larger your basic body makeup, the more servings are recommended.

Let's stop here for a second. Think about what you ate yesterday. Better yet, write it over there in the margin. Were there four to eleven servings of grain in the menu? If you answer yes, good for you. That means you are among the 12% of Americans whose diets need no improvement. If you are among the other 88%, read on.

You might wonder, "Are these recommendations the USDA's way of trying to bolster our grain markets?" That's not a bad idea, but the actual reason has to do with research evidence that confirms the following:

❂ Grains are a major source of key nutrients necessary to basic body function—carbohydrates for energy, B vitamins for nervous system function, and trace minerals such as zinc for tissue healing and growth and iron for red blood cell formation.

❂ Vitamins and minerals contained in food have greater potential benefit than those from vitamin and mineral supplements because of phytochemicals contained in the foods. These substances are produced by plants as a self-defense mechanism. Research continues to determine the exact way that the phytochemicals function, but preventive value is evident.

Besides the recommendation for 4-11 servings of grain, the guidelines also urge that at least two (of four) or 5 and one-half (of eleven) of those servings be from whole grain. Those of you who raise grains know that each portion of the grain has a function as a seed for a new

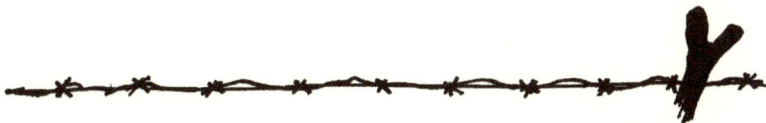

plant. The seed coat or bran, the endosperm, and the germ have protection, growth, and energy supply as their respective functions for the plant. For humans, the bran supplies fiber (you've heard the benefits of fiber by now), B vitamins and trace minerals. From the endosperm, carbohydrates and protein for energy and growth are supplied. And from the germ, antioxidant vitamin E and B vitamins are available.

Now, back to yesterday's menu that you wrote in the margin. Maybe you did better than you credited yourself for. Servings can be confusing. For example, one slice of bread is a serving. So, a sandwich with two slices is two servings. One half cup of cooked rice is a serving. I usually eat more than that when I eat rice. Do you? One tortilla is a serving. Can you stop at one? One ounce (one serving) of dry cereal is ¾ cup. Many cereal bowls are large. Filling one results in more than one serving, per serving! For more information about what makes a "serving" check labels on foods. Or on the Internet check www.health.gov/dietaryguidelines.

There's probably no way to get enough grain to satisfy a farmer. We would all like better yields. But, there is a way to satisfy your body's need for the nutrients that grain contains. Substitute grain-based snacks such as popcorn or rice cakes for non-grain snacks; serve pasta or rice instead of potatoes at half of the usual "potato meals." And where you already use grains, substitute whole grain products part of the time.

—Teddy

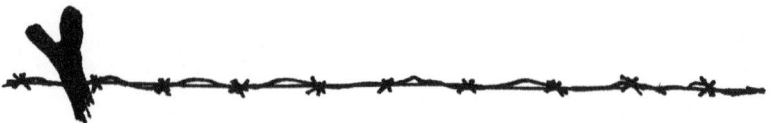

Capsule 10

A Riddle

*H*ere's a riddle. What do all of the following situations have in common?

1. You've been driving tractor for six hours, plowing your way up and down a field that seems to grow larger with every turn. You suddenly feel so sleepy that you can hardly see the guide row.

2. You're standing at the front of a room, about to speak to the Hospital Board about the need for improved emergency services.

3. That steer in the corner of the pasture has eluded all sane attempts at capture. The rest of the load is in the pen and the truck is here to haul them to auction.

4. Your oldest son announces he's set a wedding date—a happy occasion even though you didn't know he was even engaged or contemplating marriage.

5. The audience is quiet. You sit in the front row listening and silently reciting each note and word as your daughter sings her solo in the school musical.

Can you guess? At first glance, the examples don't all seem to have anything in common. Some are stressful, others are boring, some cause elation, others anxiety.

Here's the answer. In every case, you could benefit from taking a deep breath. In fact, even without "peak moments" like those, we can

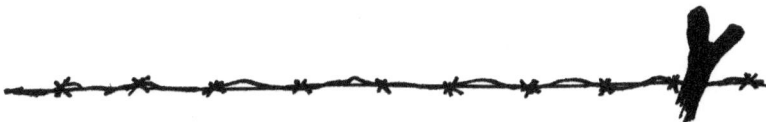

all benefit from breathing deeply, regularly.

Although breathing is automatic, many of us miss out on the benefits of using our full lung capacity because of weight, posture, habit, fatigue, anxiety and stress.

A brief review of respiration might be helpful here. The lungs are two spongy organs that sit like slightly elastic balloons inside our chests waiting to expand when the diaphragm (the muscle underneath them) expands the chest. That expansion creates negative pressure that pulls air past the nose, mouth, and trachea, down the bronchial tubes and into the lungs. The air carries oxygen to the small air sacs (alveoli) where oxygen is exchanged for carbon dioxide carried by the red blood cells. The carbon dioxide (a waste product) goes out the same way the oxygen comes in—in reverse. Under normal circumstances, that exchange helps to keep all the body tissues supplied with the oxygen they require for proper function. The exchange also helps the body's chemistry, the acid-base balance. It's all automatic when we breathe regularly. Besides creating the exchange process for oxygen, breathing helps move mucous secretions so that fluid doesn't collect in the tiny alveoli and interfere with the oxygen exchange.

But even without illness to cause problems with respiration, we often restrict our breathing. Fatigue may make us too tired to exert the effort. Poor posture can reduce the expandability of the chest. Abdominal weight can press upward and limit the downward movement of the diaphragm. And aging can reduce the elasticity of the chest wall. Stress or anxiety or even joyful excitement can make us "hold our breath." Without even realizing it, we may be breathing with only a portion of our lungs.

It's a problem that's easy to remedy. Sit or stand straight. Inhale deeply. Hold the breath for a count of eight. Exhale slowly for another eight count. Do that six or more times, slowly. Remind yourself to do that several times daily.

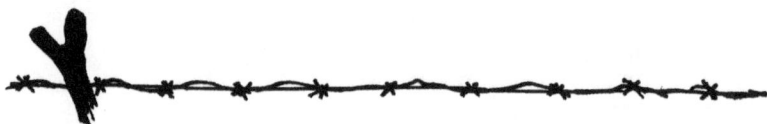

Maybe that sounds too simple to be a useful health promotion activity. Certainly it's possible to learn more complicated breathing exercises such as are included in some programs of yoga or meditation. But, I offer *simple* because even with that basic practice, several valuable results can occur.

The results? First, by improving oxygen exchange, you get increased alertness (better plowing), improved muscle function and reduced mental fatigue. The second result is relaxation and sense of calm (fewer butterflies during public speaking; ability to laugh at that hold-out steer). The third result is improved posture (every time you sit or stand tall to breathe, posture improves). And finally, there's combating the pooling of secretions in the alveoli and counteracting the age-related reduction in chest wall expandability, both of which improve alveolar respiratory function.

The best feature of all for this daily exercise is that it easily becomes a habit because the effects are positive and immediate. And it's free!

—Teddy

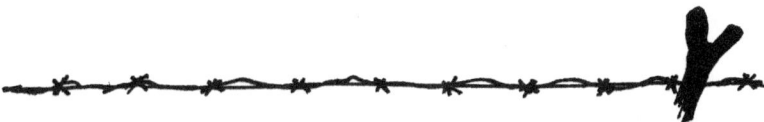

Capsule 11

Things That Take My Breath Away

*B*egging Rodgers and Hammerstein's forgiveness, I would like to list not my ten favorite things but ten things I see everyday in the country that still take my breath away.

Take time to be still and make your own list. Point out your favorite things to your children and your grandchildren. Help them develop their senses by modeling your appreciation and awareness. By design, we have been given five senses. Use them all and enjoy this wonderful world.

Finally, be glad this is a book, not a musical, and you only have to read my list and not listen to me sing it. But if you feel like running around on top of a mountain, whirling in circles, ala Julie Andrews, go for it. Doing that will probably take your breath away, too!

- ☻ Fireflies at night
- ☻ Spider webs (though not the spiders)
- ☻ Double rainbows
- ☻ Unbridled horses running through the field
- ☻ Driving my neighbor's 1950 Chevy pick-up
- ☻ Raindrops on roses, on the pavement, on anything
- ☻ Litters of piglets

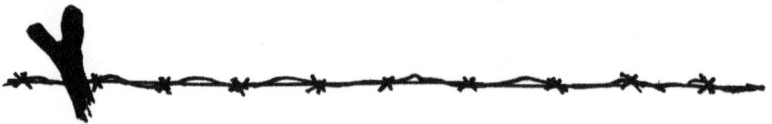

- ✪ Harvest moon rising over the football field on an October Friday night
- ✪ Deer jumping the fence
- ✪ A West Texas sunset

—Sue Jane

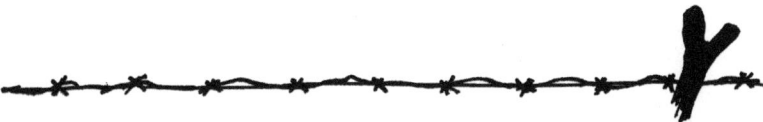

Capsule 12

Gimme One of Those

*T*he word is that the name "gimme cap" originated the first time an enterprising dealer decided to use the previously blank front piece on a billed cap for advertising. As the hats were handed out to customers providing lots of walking billboards, the wearers were heard to say, "Yeah, old Charlie gimme this cap when I bought my seed from him this year." Millions of those billed creations have all but replaced fully brimmed hats for both casual and outdoor work wear. They are a great idea for advertising and a good way for the "givee" to get free headgear. But, they can be a hazard to the health of those farm and ranch people who wear them. No, I don't mean that your hair will have a permanent crease in the back. That happens when a person wears a cap, but I don't consider it a health hazard. I realize that fewer women than men wear those caps, but perhaps you can have some influence on the men who do if you have the facts.

The problem is that caps don't cast any shade on the ears and the back of the neck. Those two spots are among the most common sites for skin cancers. All of us are susceptible to sun damage and to skin cancer. The fairer the complexion, the higher the risk. Neither the damage that is evident as wrinkling or spotting nor skin cancer happens in a day. It is the accumulated effect of repeated exposure that causes the problem.

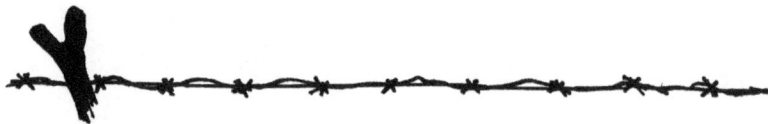

Every day, the sunlight beams ultraviolet rays on any exposed skin. And over time, the damage occurs.

While wrinkling and spotting are annoying signs of our years and our sun exposure, they are not as dangerous as skin cancers. The three most common skin cancers are basal cell carcinoma, squamous cell carcinoma, and malignant melanoma. The first two types are more common in people over 40 years of age, but melanoma often affects young people. Melanoma and squamous cell carcinoma may spread beyond the original site to other organs. Therefore, they are the more dangerous types of skin cancers. But, even if the basal cell cancers are less dangerous and usually do not metastasize, for the 400,000 or so new cases each year in the U.S., they are no fun either. Just ask anyone who has had a piece of the ear or nose "whittled" to remove one if they enjoyed the procedure.

What can you do about skin cancer if you do not plan to stay indoors all the time? There are two approaches that we should each use regularly. One is inspection and the other is preventive action. Neither one takes much time or any special training. But, they do mean taking on new habits. Let me explain. Inspecting our own skin in detail is something that most of us haven't done since we were teenagers. But, making a habit of a thorough once over once a month can be an important part of identifying any suspicious spots. Here's what to look for:

- A raised, thickened area, usually small, on a sun-exposed surface, lasting more than a week.
- An area such as described above that bleeds easily and/or appears scaly.
- A raised pearly colored nodule with small blood vessels (spidery looking) on the surface and a rolled appearing edge.

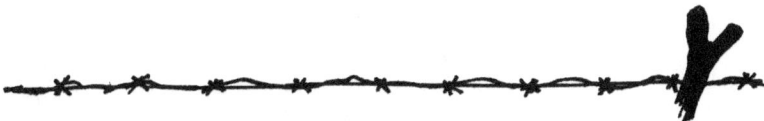

❂ A mole or freckle that is irregularly shaped, with irregular borders, that is larger than the end of the little finger, and that has variegated color or has changed color.

Unless you have a good long mirror, you may have to have a helper to examine your back, but don't skip that part. It is important. The benefit of inspecting the skin once a month is that you are likely to notice changes early as you notice differences from one month to the next.

So, with that new habit on board, you are ready to think about preventive actions. The choices are three. First, stay indoors. That's not very realistic, though. We all work outside a great deal of the time. The next two actions are a bit more likely to be acceptable. Covering up is a good strategy. That means wearing long sleeves and reserving shorts for special leisure occasions, preferably not during the peak sun periods between 10 a.m. and 4 p.m. daily. Even with covering clothing, that leaves the backs of the hands, the face, ears and neck exposed. And for some folks whose hair has "gone South", the top of the head is a danger spot as well. So, sunscreen is a must have item. Choose one with a sun protection factor (SPF) rating no less than 15. Apply it liberally and remember to repeat it during the day.

A wide brimmed hat is the best choice of headgear. It gives added protection to the ears, nose and back of the neck and shades the eyes. But, I doubt that we are likely to see the disappearance of the billed cap any time soon. So, here's an idea. The next time someone offers you a new "gimme cap," say "Sure, thanks a lot, and are you going to "gimme" a bottle of sunscreen to go with it?" Maybe we can start a new trend in advertising—sunscreen with the logo of your favorite implement company on it. And maybe we can start another trend—a decline in the number of skin cancers.

—Teddy

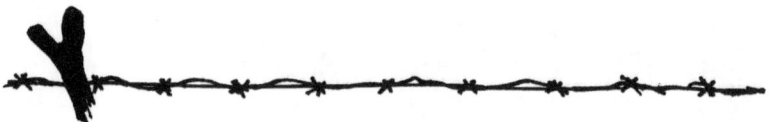

Capsule 13

From Dusk to Dawn

*I*n the American Southwest, the summer hours between 8 p.m. and 6 a.m. qualify for the phrase, "dusk to dawn", give or take a time zone or two. Many people associated with agriculture live the adage, "make hay while the sun shines." But I'm not a farmer, and it is as the sun sets and after that I like to make hay.

Dusk to dawn is prime time for doing some things that might just enhance your work as a farm or ranch woman. Here are some suggestions for things to do after the other folks at your place go to bed and before they rise.

First of all, consider the decreased risk of skin cancer. Those bad ultraviolet rays are just about gone as dusk nears, so toss that floppy hat, lose the long sleeves, and enjoy the fresh air. Go as bare as you dare. Sit on the porch, preferably in the dark, and chill. It's not weird. It's money saved by not having to buy sunscreen.

Another suggestion involves the family, perhaps your small children or grandchildren. Nocturnal nature appreciation is so important these days—kids need to step away from those video games and get outside. It's what varmints do at night. They frolic. They're frisky. Go on a hike or pickup truck ride with the kiddies. Look for deer, jack rabbits, and my favorite, tarantulas.

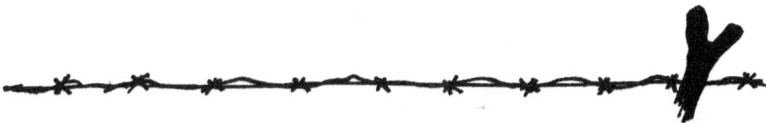

When she was younger, my daughter Julie actually formed a Tarantula Club, sort of like an Audubon Society for Arachnophiles. She and her friends would gather at dusk to see how many they could find. They would stalk the spiders. When successful, the girls would talk one of the dads into letting one or two crawl up his arm. Cheap family fun. The extra money saved on entertainment allowed one family to buy a blender to make margaritas.

My personal favorite dusk to dawn activity involves the constellations. Star-gazing is great in the country because you don't have the urban lights to obscure how magnificently heavenly orbs light up our world.

In 1986, Halley's Comet was making its once-in-every-76 years appearance. I dragged Julie, then four, out of bed several nights in a row to witness history. I just knew this was as important as her first tooth, her first steps, her first solid food. Surely there was a space in the baby book for first comet. She thought we were hunting for tarantulas and so was eager to join me, at least on the first night. Once she discovered it was some "dumb ol" comet passing this way, she was not amused. I think she fell asleep in the car as we drove to the edge of town to see Halley, but I sure got a good view of its streaking magic and felt I had done my job as a parent.

Of course, some folks want to do other extracurricular activities from dusk to dawn. I don't mean to be a party pooper, but aren't my suggestions more cost efficient, safer, and well, innocent? Cover charges are non-existent. If you must kick up your heels in the country, what was once called a hootenanny (the politically correct term is barn dance) can be revived and with a profit.

While everyone else is sleeping soundly, rent out the barn to urban dwellers looking for an alternative club setting. Barns are usually some distance from the main house, so others should continue to snooze. If you live in a wet county, sell some of those distilled spirits. I would

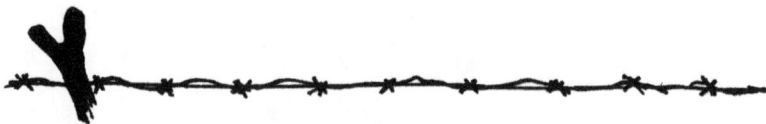

suggest you designate drivers, however, as people who live in the city don't understand dirt road driving when they are sober, much less when they aren't.

You won't have much overhead. A bouncer can be provided cheap. That's what a bull is for, so this will lead to increased profits for the farm or ranch. Your husband will be so proud of you and want to reward you with a trip to Las Vegas.

And we all know what you can do there from dusk to dawn.

—Sue Jane

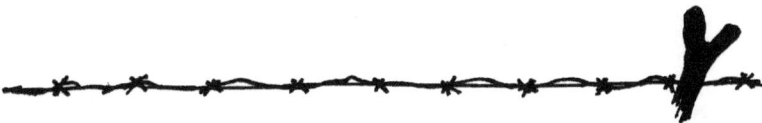

Capsule 14

What's Not To Love?

I found some health advice that does all of the following:

- ◎ offers the possibility of benefiting agriculture
- ◎ is easy, even pleasurable to follow
- ◎ is based on well-designed research
- ◎ suggests a possibility of decreasing the risks of developing Type II diabetes

What's not to love about that kind of advice? Nothing, as far as I can see. Let me tell you about it.

Sorting through research reports from 2002, I spied a title that included the words "nuts and peanut butter consumption and risk of Type II diabetes in women."

"Oh, no," I thought. "Now I have to avoid peanut butter, give up almonds, eschew cashews! Settle down," I advised myself. "Maybe that's not what this is about."

Much to my relief, I read that my peanut butter-for-breakfast might even be good for me. The research was conducted on 83,818 women from 11 states over a 16-year period in the Nurses' Health Study. Those were women aged 34 to 59 when the research began. After 16 years, in that group, 3206 new cases of Type II diabetes were diagnosed. Statistical

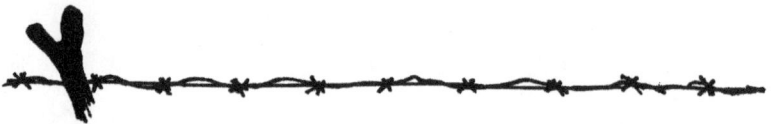

analysis showed a significant difference in reduced risk of that disease in women who ate nuts or peanut butter. The risk declined as the consumption rose. The categories were nut consumption never/almost never; < 1 time per week; 1–4 times per week; and > 5 times per week. A large number of other possible factors for the relationship were ruled out. They included intake of fat and cereal fiber. The relationship persisted across different categories of age, Body Mass Index, family history of diabetes, smoking and alcohol consumption.

If you are interested in reading the study, it's in the *Journal of the American Medical Association*, 2002, pages 2554–2560.

So, the research was sound and the conclusion was logical. The researchers *did not* prove that nuts prevent diabetes. But they did show that there was a relationship between eating nuts and reduced risk of developing Type II diabetes. Neither did they know why the relationship of more nuts = less diabetes, but it did. In addition, nuts are a source of trace minerals and vitamin E along with some protein. If you are a person who, because of high blood pressure or other condition should watch sodium in your diet, the unsalted variety should be your choice. The salt would easily use up your daily allotment of sodium.

Good enough for a nut lover like me. Here's a way I can increase consumption of production grown in our region. Peanuts, pecans, and pistachios are immediate candidates. Let's see. I'll eat the suggested one ounce and just to be really helpful I'll do it every day. That's 365 ounces or 22.75 pounds per year. I'd be doing my part.

But wait, what about those calories? Nuts are calorie dense as well as nutrient dense. A one-ounce serving of nuts (about ¼ cup of nut meats or 2 tablespoons of peanut butter) is around 130–150 calories. Though they are high in fat, the fat is the polyunsaturated "good fat." So, the real issue is the increased calories.

The easiest way to deal with that is to make a substitute—the nuts for something not as beneficial. The researchers suggest trading

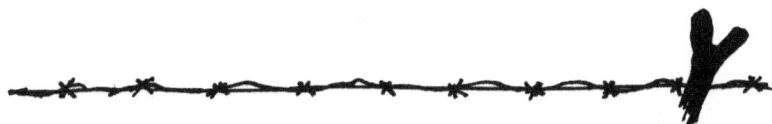

them for processed meat or refined grain products like donuts or cake.

Another way of keeping the nuts without major calorie increase is to eat the nuts without attaching them to other foods. With that in mind, avoid making pralines or pecan pie the source of nuts. Pistachios direct from the shell would trump those included in shortbread cookies. And peanuts in a candy bar are less desirable than a no-frills handful. Incidentally, a palmful is just about the recommended ¼ cup serving.

If you're a real peanut butter fan, you'll know there's nothing wrong with unadorned peanut butter eaten straight from the jar. I personally have a variety of favored serving implements for this treat. There's a spoon, a knife, or when I'm in a hurry (gotta have some peanut butter NOW), my index finger.

You might ask if men can benefit from nut consumption as well as women. As the research only studied women, I have no authoritative answer about men. But, I'm willing to share the peanut butter.

—Teddy

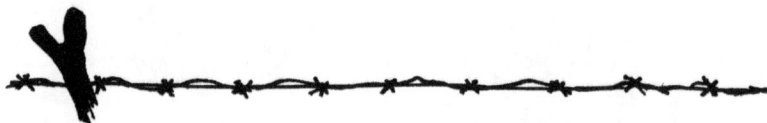

Capsule 15

Food for Thought

*T*hinking and eating are two of my favorite things so I'm really an expert on the expression "here's some food for thought."

When I was a teenager, there were foods that, in my opinion, were not edible in any form. Asparagus, liver, squash, meat loaf, carrots, and tomatoes made my top ten Worst Foods List year after year.

Then, my taste buds matured—probably a post-adolescence thing.

After much thought (of course), I have come to the conclusion that developing a taste for those previous yucky-but-good-for-you foods is a sign of growing up.

When we're young, there are several factors that influence our decisions. One, the more our parents force an issue, the more likely we are to resist. So, "eat your vegetables" becomes a parental mantra that goes down the wrong way.

Two, when young, we think we know more than we do, i.e., asparagus must be gross because it smells and looks gross. We aren't experimental with anything other than the big three: sex, music, and alcohol/tobacco. I only smoked a cigar once, I grew up with the Carpenters and the Beatles, and I won't comment on the other because my parents are still living.

But, there's no one telling me now what I have to eat, and my world isn't so limited anymore.

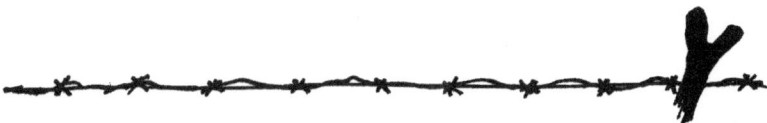

I've traveled to Boston and eaten clam chowder, to the Northwest and had some of the best fresh fruit pies that exist on the planet, and to Louisiana, famous for their great meat pies and gumbo.

Maybe I just had to grow up a little or maybe it was having to eat my own cooking that made me learn to like different kinds of foods. It could also be attributed to my mother-in-law's cooking which was wonderful and free and done in her kitchen, not mine. She could make asparagus as delectable to me as angel food cake. At her house, I fell in love with fried squash.

It has occurred to me, too, that many of my other "tastes" have been broadened the older I get. Once, libraries were nothing to me but places to do term papers. Amazingly enough, I go there now to get books to read—for fun! Our small town doesn't have a county library, but the facility at school works just fine for some good reading material. At night I'll go up and sit in some comfortable chairs and catch up on my newspaper reading and get my weekly magazine fix.

When I was younger, buying new was mandatory—from cars to clothes. I was determined to do away with that hand-me-down thing that my mother grew up with on the farm. Today, I am working to save money, not for retirement and travel but for a '55 Chevy truck. I bowl in my dad's old bowling shirt with his insurance agency sponsor still stitched above the pocket. I wear overalls and flip flops and my aunt's old 1970s sunglasses.

So here's some food for thought for both parents and their children. Be patient with each other. Don't make the table or the clothing or the vehicle a battleground. Tastes will change soon enough.

As for the original remarks made about food, if you're under 18, enjoy those fast fried foods. You'll find out soon enough that they can give you high cholesterol.

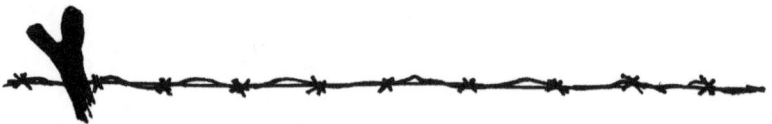

If your taste buds and every other part of your body are well past ripe, unclog them with healthy things. I suggest fruit, and every time I order a hot fudge sundae at the local Dairy Queen, I ask for a cherry on top.

—Sue Jane

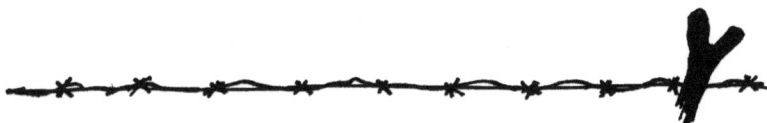

Capsule 16

In Praise of Toothpicks

*T*he reclining dental chair tipped me so that I was staring at the ceiling. I couldn't avoid the poster that had been placed in what was now my line of sight. What I was compelled to read was "floss regularly"—more of a command than an encouragement.

The hygienist approached. Just before she put her equipment into my mouth, I managed to ask, "What about toothpicks?"

"Toothpicks are fine," she responded, smiling behind her mask. (I couldn't *see* her smile, but her eyes crinkled behind her protective lenses. I preferred to believe she was smiling rather than sneering at the thought of *toothpicks.*)

Please don't get me wrong. I have nothing against floss. In fact, there are lots of good reasons for using it. First, it clears particles of food from the spaces between the teeth and prevents it from getting beneath the gums. The cleaning helps to prevent decay by reducing the growth medium for bacteria that cause dental caries.

Second, the stimulation of the cleansing function encourages circulation in the gums. The gums have a network of tiny capillaries that bring blood to nourish these tissues. If the circulation is poor, this encourages gingivitis—gum inflammation and infection. These capillaries are just below the surface. If the gums are healthy and the circulation is

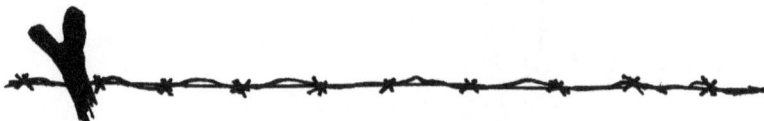

good, they don't bleed. But, if you notice that the gums are puffy, red and bleed easily, take action.

Are you cleaning both teeth and gums regularly? Gentle salt-water rinses can help restore gum integrity if there is just a single spot that is bleeding. But if it is widespread or does not heal readily, a visit to the dentist is in order. Bleeding gums may not only signal gum disease, but also can be a sign of systemic problems. For example, a vitamin deficiency may prompt the bleeding or there may be some other illness affecting the ability of the blood to clot. Or, cigarette smoking may have affected the capillaries. Take a look. Are your gums a healthy pink, are they puffy and red, are they pale and receding? If they are pale, that can be a sign of anemia. In any case, the first response to unhealthy looking gums should be to check that they are clean and regularly stimulated.

That leads me back to the toothpick question. It seems to me that toothpicks are far more likely to be the tool of choice for between-brushing cleaning and stimulation than is floss. My reasons? Well, for one thing, they are free. Unless you want to buy toothpicks, you can come by them in almost any dining establishment. Take several.

I take that back. Not *all* eateries offer toothpicks. Some upscale places ignore the fact that toothpicks are a cultural fixture—at least in a lot of rural areas. Upon dining in one of these spots, you may need to do what my grandfather was fond of doing—whittle one. Or, you can take out your Swiss Army Knife and use the one so neatly included in the handle.

I mentioned the toothpick as a cultural fixture. By that I mean that it is accepted as a part of one's gear in many segments of society. I guess that one shouldn't have a toothpick in sight while in an evening gown, but you will see one in eight of ten mouths leaving the numerous all-you-can-eat buffets around here. That's a far higher number than those who floss at the table.

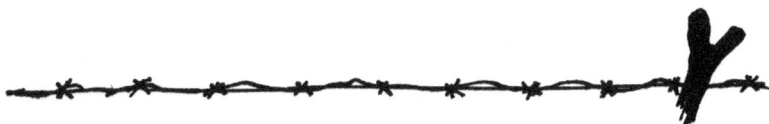

Also noteworthy is that a toothpick only requires one hand to operate. Floss takes two. Yet another point in favor of the sacred splinter.

While toothpicks do well at the cleaning and gum stimulating function, they perform another function that floss never could. They are good for dealing with tension. Long after its more common use is served, the toothpick is there, in the corner of the mouth, available to be chewed on, to use as punctuation, and to occupy the hands in stressful moments.

Sometimes we even forget they are there. I heard a story about a Texan (okay, a West Texan) who had worked hard to get the grades and entrance exam scores needed to be accepted to one of the health professional schools. It seems that he turned up for his interview in his best suit with a toothpick in his mouth—which stayed there throughout the interview. Only the culturally competent interviewer would recognize that no disrespect was intended. The young man was just being himself, good gums and all. That he was admitted to the school is testament to the fact that toothpicks are superior to floss for lots of occasions. Try to imagine the tangle he would have had if he had flossed his way through the interview!

—Teddy

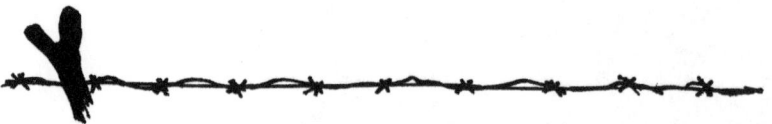

Capsule 17

Stretching Again

*F*lexibilility. That's what I'm pursuing. As is my routine, I'm down on the floor stretching, watched attentively and occasionally joined by Pete Jones, the fast white dog. Later, I use the same excuse (maintaining flexibility) as I put first one and then the other foot up on the kitchen cabinet and bend to try to touch my head to my knee. I'll never be a ballerina, but I don't intend to be a stiff old gal either.

I'll use that same reason as I give myself a break from "today's list" and work a crossword puzzle. I couldn't have been more pleased when I read recently that working crossword puzzles is one way to maintain *mental* flexibility, another important aspect of good health.

What a treat it is when something you enjoy doing is also good for your health. Besides crossword puzzles, other mental activity suggested included reading, taking classes, talking with other people, going to museums, listening to radio and watching television. The suggestions came from an article aimed at those in their middle years who hope to stay physically, mentally and emotionally healthy as they age. A key point was that it's better to begin mentally stimulating activities early (or continue them from youth) to cultivate the habit so that declines in function are reduced or prevented as we grow older. Rather than saying "I can't remember anything anymore," we should engage in those activities that require us to "use it" rather than "lose it." Make a game of

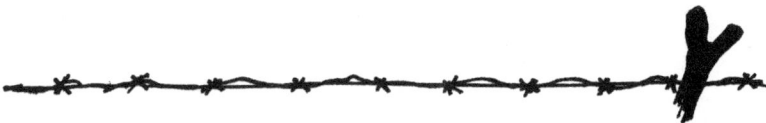

memorizing and recalling lists—any list will do—books of the Bible, names of the states and their capitols, items to buy at the grocery store. Memory is only one function that maintains or improves with practice. Computation skills are another. Exercise that by balancing the checkbook without using a calculator. Good advice.

As I thought more about maintaining mental abilities, I realized that skill or strength is one thing and flexibility is another. Just as with the muscles and joints, stretching means pushing a little bit to stay elastic. In addition to mental strengthening, we need to stretch also.

I saw a newspaper story about a 94 year-old woman who's running for the Senate in New Hampshire. She's not satisfied to be aware of issues and form an opinion. She's taking action. I know a man of 90 + years who took a course to learn Spanish last year. A 50 year-old woman is learning to create computer spreadsheets. She'll use that skill in her volunteer work at the local library. Each one of those is good mental exercise and something of a stretch.

There are lots of ways adults can stretch their mental abilities. Think of the following categories of "mental stretching" activities:

- Learn a new skill.
- Practice an old skill and put it to a new use.
- Intentionally encounter new ideas.

Learn a new skill. This offers lots of possibilities. I'll mention a few and hope you'll add others. Learn to play a new game. If you've played dominoes as a youngster, try 42. If cooking is something you love, challenge yourself to develop new recipes. Learn to play a musical instrument. Try drawing or painting. Computers offer plenty of opportunities. You can develop web pages, trace genealogy and create graphics. If you're learning a new skill or adding to an old one, you're stretching.

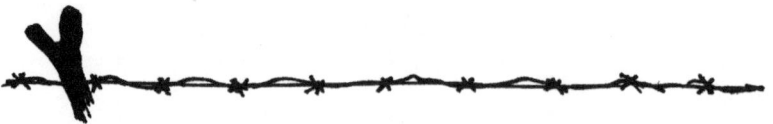

Put an old skill to a new use. A person who has raised cattle could learn about training cattle dogs. It's animal care put to a new use. If you've always been good at repairing small appliances, try building a lamp. Are you a reader? Write a book review or a discussion guide for the next one you enjoy. The stretch is in going from just enjoying the book to analyzing it and communicating your ideas.

Intentionally encounter new ideas. Talk with people you don't ordinarily spend time with. Is the new clerk at the convenience store interested in the County Commissioner election? Start a discussion. Listen to a different radio station as you plow. Argue with the talk radio host. Search the Internet or visit the library to find information on subjects that you hear or see on television. Discuss what you find with anyone who'll hold still.

None of us relishes the idea of mental decline for ourselves or our loved ones. Whatever your age, begin now to do mental stretching. Who knows what you might be capable of at 90? There's always the County Commissioner's race.

—Teddy

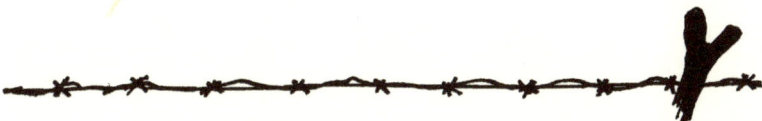

Capsule 18

Share the Wealth

*T*he gifted.

They are our reminders on Earth that God can do truly remarkable things with mere mortals. How else can a boy write a composition at age seven or attempt to compose an opera by ten?

Samuel Barber was arguably the United States' equivalent of Mozart. His music is as lyrical and inspired as any words a person might read from Scripture. God had his hand in this composer's work. His church or choice or his faith I do not know. I do know that something like Barber's "Adagio for Strings" can only come from the Giver of the gift.

Most gifts are not as pronounced. We may not profit financially or become famous for our talents. Still, we are all gifted.

The word is not an adjective to describe ourselves. It is a verb— an action verb—telling what a higher being had done *for* us and *to* us. He gifts us.

He gives to us the ability to say kind things sincerely, to smile at just the right time, to sew, to quilt, to cook, to play sports, to repair machinery, to love purely, to love those hard to love, to write, to draw, to comfort, to laugh, and to make others laugh, to take photographs and capture moments, to organize, to paint, to be loving grandmothers, to be patient, to sing, to shun gossip, to listen, to impart wisdom, to make

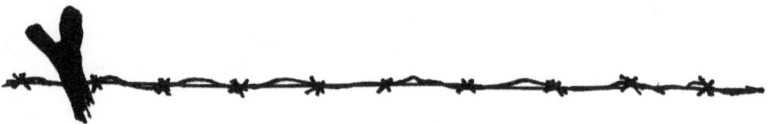

a timely phone call, to be nice to telemarketers, to speak in public, to care for the elderly, to care.

Surely out of all the gifts that are showered upon us, we can find one to use in our homes or our communities to make life better for ourselves and those around us. The inspiration to write a beautiful adagio is rare thing, but in abundance are the daily gifts mentioned above.

If we so choose to use them, we can leave people humming a melody they will never forget.

—Sue Jane

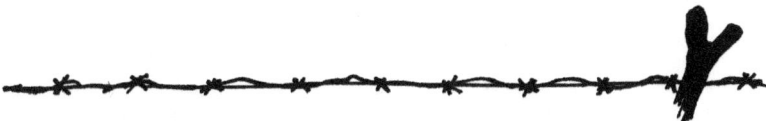

Capsule 19

Why Worry?

"*I*'ve been having trouble sleeping lately." "Have you? Me too, I've been worrying about the weather."

I was eavesdropping on a conversation at the post office. Since I've promised myself not to worry about things I cannot change, including the weather and the economy, what that set me thinking about was sleep. No, I did not rush home for a nap—what I did was make a list of things that interrupt or delay sleep. Before I show you my list, I will tell you why it is important to know about disturbed sleep.

You will probably say that I have a good grasp of the obvious when I say that *reduced* hours of sleep lead to fatigue. Not so obvious is the effect of *interruptions* of sleep. Both reduced hours of sleep and interrupted (even if typically sufficient hours) sleep can produce fatigue, can aggravate chronic pain, can diminish the function of the immune system, and can make you a cranky and unpleasant person. Each of those problems has results of its own.

Fatigue diminishes productivity and discourages enjoyment of all aspects of life. Chronic pain reduces function and encourages increased medication use which, in turn, can cause problems due to drug side effects. The immune system of a poorly rested person is less able to respond competently to infectious organisms. Irritability caused

by reduced or interrupted sleep can result in bad relationships and family discord.

When sleep disruptions are only occasional, we usually overcome the difficulty by catching up with a couple of early-to-bed nights. When sleep disruption continues, the troubles creep in.

Adults typically need seven to nine hours of sleep regardless of age, although after about age 60, some small reduction in need is seen. So, a person who once regularly slept eight hours may only feel a need for seven and a half total hours as she ages. The other important part is getting the necessary amount of the different levels of sleep. The sleep stages are from light to heavy (stages 1-4) and stage 5 which is Rapid Eye Movement (REM) Sleep, when dreaming occurs. Good quality sleep that provides the rest an adult needs must have all of those stages, with about 20% being REM Sleep, regardless of age. Sleep comes in cycles, going from light to heavy (stages 1-4) and back to lighter (stages 3 and 2) and then to REM. "Restarts" because of interruptions can mean missing out on the necessary REM sleep. For that reason, uninterrupted sleep is most restful.

Here's the list of causes that I came up with. You can make additions by recalling "what kept you up" most recently.

- Children. Infants and young children cry, are sick, need to be fed, and sometimes just wake their parents for company. "Hi, I'm ready to play, even if it is two a.m." Older children have dates, drive cars, play on ball teams that travel and other things that tend to keep parents awake.
- Irrigation motors. Irrigation motors are not the only farm or ranch equipment that may need tending in the middle of the night. Any machinery that you set the alarm to go out to check on qualifies.
- Pain. Chronic pain from ailments like arthritis seems more acute

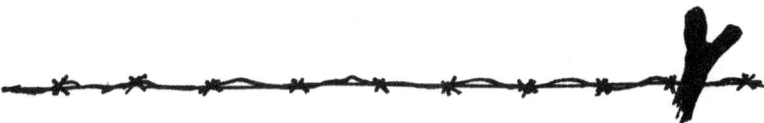

at night, at least in part because of fatigue from the day's activity and partly because there are fewer distractions to take the mind off of the pain.

- ✿ Bathroom visits. Waking to urinate is a common sleep disturber.
- ✿ Animal births. Birthing season for your livestock can be pretty hectic. You know that not all difficult births occur at night, but it sure seems so.
- ✿ Alcohol, caffeine, and tobacco. Caffeine and tobacco are stimulants that may delay the onset of sleep. Alcohol, on the other hand, acts as a sedative and may, in small amounts encourage the onset of sleep. In large amounts, the effect is different. At first, sleep may come, but the alcohol suppresses REM Sleep, so the effect is disruption of the sleep cycle, thus poor rest.
- ✿ Worry. Having trouble turning off thoughts can upset sleep. Thinking at bedtime is a little like entertaining guests. You have to be careful whom you invite, and you need to have a sure-fire way to get them to leave.

There's probably not a lot to be done about the sleep that children cause us to lose except to share the load when possible and try to take naps. The same goes for irrigation motors and animal births.

But, you can deal with the other sleep villains. Pain should be treated particularly well at bedtime. Whatever medicine and/or other tactic works for the pain should be used regularly just before bedtime. The bathroom visits may be a habit—you wake from stage 1 or 2 sleep, so you go to the bathroom. If you don't really need to go, don't! Close your eyes and lie quietly. Sleep may return. Or, you may have a urinary tract problem. An infection is often the culprit in a female's urinary tract. In a male, it might be an enlarged prostate or an infection. If habit is not the cause, get yourself checked by your health care provider. If you are in the bathroom because you take a diuretic, take it earlier in the day so

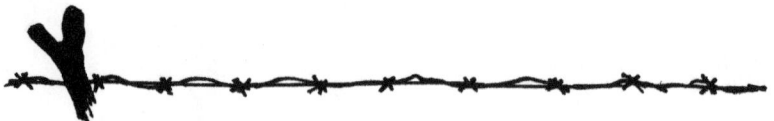

it does not keep you up. Moderation or abstinence will eliminate the alcohol, caffeine and tobacco problems.

As for worry, there's always plenty to think about and to allow to become constant visitors—worries. I will tell you more about stress reduction, including reducing worrying, later. For now, just promise me you will do what I plan to do about the weather—not worry about it. I plan to sleep as well as I can every night and wake up rested and ready for whatever comes.

—Teddy

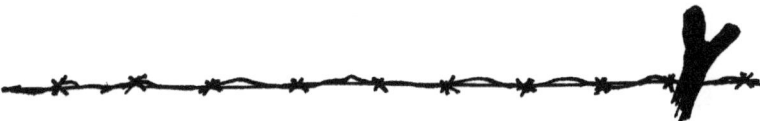

Capsule 20

Sweet Dreams

*B*efore I die, there's one thing I really want to do other than visit Yankee Stadium.

I want to sleep in a barn.

My parents would respond with skepticism because I was their child that was deathly afraid of spiders, snakes, scorpions, thunderstorms, and grass burrs—things I could not escape in the West Texas countryside.

Even when I read *Charlotte's Web*, I couldn't get past the creepiness of an eight-legged creature, kind as she was, spinning those word webs. Why didn't someone take his or her boots off and smash her?

My transformation to adventurer came late in life. I divorced at 38, and it was like a magic wand was waved and poof! All paranoias and phobias disappeared.

I began to travel by airplane again, sleep through brilliant lightning storms, and laugh rather than scream at spiders and scorpions stuck on those sticky pads hidden behind the washer and dryer.

I'm not sure where the slumber-party-in-the-barn idea came from, but I am somehow convinced that it would represent something important. Some people have first communions, others have bar or bat mitzvahs, and those cotillion belles have debuts. Why can't a middle-aged woman from the country have a sleepover in a barn?

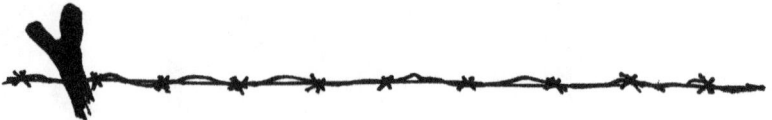

Uninterrupted sleep is crucial to anyone's health, but let's face it. Women in their late forties and early fifties are going through hell. Our metabolism is stuck. We go to the bathroom at night more than we do during the day. Hot flashes hit like tsunamis. It's not pretty.

After the dutiful years of childbirth and fulfilling the roles we were assigned by Eve's blunder, I think one night in a barn is a small thing for which to ask.

My mom said that she never got to sleep in the barn; that was what the boys got to do. So, another reason why I want to do this is for my mother and for all the other women her age who were denied this right on the basis of their gender.

What has started as a simple wish for sweet dreams in a pastoral setting has become my crusade for all women everywhere. Why not? We are women. Hear us snore.

With a good night's rest, I can handle anything. Even a spider that spells out "menopause."

—Sue Jane

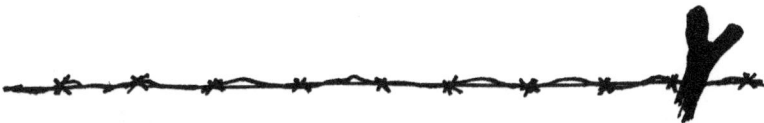

Capsule 21

Make or Break, It's Up To You

You've heard it said, I'm sure, "It's a make or break deal." Maybe the topic was planting cotton when the market was volatile. It could have been buying a pen of cattle at the local feed yard. Or maybe it was that "sure thing" you heard about ratite ranching because steaks from flightless birds were going to replace beef as our red meat of choice. Whatever the topic, the message was clear: you could win or lose. Big.

"Make or break" causes me to think of something else. That something is habits, in particular, the habits that affect our health. Now you're probably expecting me to launch into telling you about breaking some bad habits. I could. We all have some bad ones we need to break—like dipping snuff or eating too many fried foods. But, I won't. I prefer to be positive, to focus on making new habits. "Sure, take the easy way," you say. Actually though, making new habits is just about as difficult as breaking old ones. Researchers say it takes about six months of working at it to make a new habit. The fact is that changing our behavior is never a snap.

Think about the suggestions you've heard or read—doing stretching exercises, drinking more fluid, using sunscreen, and wearing a mask for respiratory protection, for example. Each of those involves making a new habit. To get from "thinking about doing it" to actually habitually doing any of those requires more than just agreeing with me

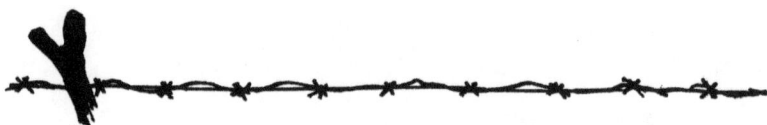

that it is a good idea. An important part of making any one of those things a positive habit is to make it convenient.

Here is a little story about how convenience can encourage making a new habit. We have a friend in Friona. Sounds like a song title, doesn't it?. In fact, he's such a good friend that he puts up with my giving him health advice. This friend—let's call him John—works very hard, early to late. Seldom eating breakfast and often skipping lunch, he works cattle. Now he sees that the cattle eat regularly. Anyway, you get the picture. Well, John needed to take some medicine for a couple of weeks to help some tendonitis he had. I was quick to point out that he should take it three times during the day with food. How to make that convenient, I wondered, for a man whose morning ration was mostly coffee. Maybe if he gets in the habit, he would eat more regularly even after the medicine taking was finished, I thought.

It was then that the Ag-Pack was invented. Okay, it's not an invention. The Ag-Pack is an assembly of things that make some healthy habits convenient. It is particularly for farm and ranch people, hence the name. Picture this. Take a flip-top cooler of about the 8 by 12 inch size. (The Igloo Little Playmate works well, but any similar cooler will do.) Put in the following items:

- ✪ A one-quart water bottle—a rigid nalgene camper's canteen with a screw-on attached top is good. Fill it with cold water.
- ✪ One small cold pack of the type that can be refrozen daily.
- ✪ A small plastic bottle (like vitamins come in) with enough powdered sports drink (Gatorade works well) to make an 8 ounce serving when water is added.
- ✪ A plastic bag into which you "zip" the following: At least two "nutrition dense" breakfast bars. (You can use your own favorite quick breakfast items instead. For example, take two large oatmeal cookies and make a peanut butter sandwich of them. Or if there is a good cook at your house, take two homemade

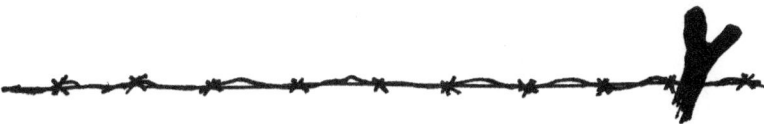

granola bars.) The idea is to have some easy to eat breakfast item available. Some hard candy or some small sweets for when you need a quick boost. Chewing gum. A piece of fruit.

- A sandwich if you are not likely to get away for lunch.

Make a drawstring bag out of some fabric piece that you have handy. (John's is heavy khaki twill I had in the closet.) Thread a long boot lace through the top for a drawstring. (The bootlace will be used to tie the bag to the cooler. It will also come in handy if you ever need to deliver a baby on a turnrow—tie off the umbilical cord.)
In the drawstring pouch, place these items:

- Some adhesive bandages. The number you need depends on how often you cut or scrape yourself.
- One paper mask
- One container of sunscreen—SPF more than 30
- One container of insect repellent
- One container of antibiotic skin ointment such as Neosporin
- One pill bottle with several ibuprofen or acetaminophen tablets and a few antihistamine tablets
- Any prescription medicine that you need to take during the day

Every morning, put in a fresh bottle of water and a frozen cold pack. Check that the other items are replaced if you have used them. Put that neat little assembly in the pickup seat next to you. That's your Ag-Pack.

In John's case, he just needed to reach in after he fed the calves and take a minute to eat the breakfast bars. Then he could take his pills. In your case, with an Ag-Pack, you might find it more convenient to get in the two-quart minimum of water each day or to put on a mask when

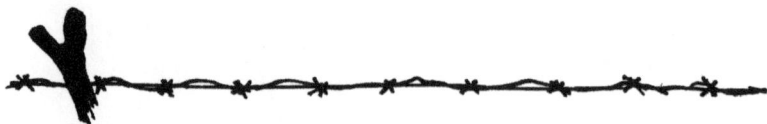

you shovel grain. If you are a woman who chooses not to shovel grain or to work with the animals very often, your Ag-Pack may not see daily use. That's fine. It will wait patiently on a shelf for the days when you do. It will be ready to help you make or keep some good health habits.

With an Ag-Pack, at least four good habits are easier to make: eating regularly to keep up energy, increasing fluid intake, using sunscreen, and wearing a mask to protect the respiratory tract. It helps with making the habits because it is convenient. Convenience improves the chance of making new behavior become habit. Maybe it's not emu ranching, but habits are definitely "make or break" as far as good health is concerned.

—Teddy

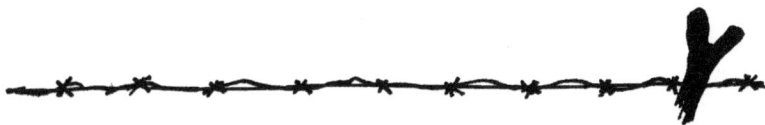

Capsule 22

Write On!

I was a working mother.

Of course, every mother is a working mother, but let's don't worry about political correctness. Everybody knows what the phrase means, and I was one of "them." But even I got a few things right when it came to maternal effort, and my Monday night letter-writing with my daughters was one such endeavor.

The girls were probably nine and four—Julie, the oldest, had recently learned to write cursive. Since that was a new thing to her, I seized her eagerness to write while it lasted. My four-year old liked to color, so her correspondence included a crayon creation and a printed E M I L Y. To really capture my audience, we also made Monday night cookie-baking night. It was one of the cleverest things I ever came up with in the challenging world of motherhood.

Each week the girls had to write someone different. It could be and often was a relative. As a child, I had great pen-pal relationships with my mother's sisters; my daughters took that a generation further much to the delight of my Aunt Eula and Aunt Bert who both lived in Washington state. Sometimes letters were sent to cousins or family friends.

Much to my regret, I never made copies of the letters for tangible evidence of our one year of correspondence and cookies, but the memories have cookie prints and eraser smudges all over them. Today,

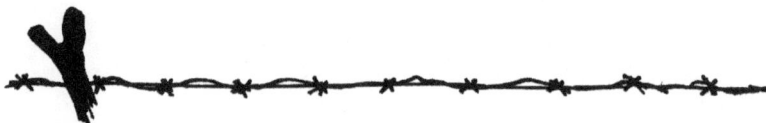

both daughters never have to be reminded to write a thank you, and often on their own sit down and write letters just because—which is the best reason of all.

Being isolated is a side effect of sorts when living in a rural community. Staying in touch takes effort. My mother taught me that as I witnessed her and her siblings remain close through their adult years. Distance was not an issue as long as there was a stamp to be bought. Stationery and postage were often gifts in our home, and they were put to good use.

Living in cities and towns accommodates friendship and kinship because personal contact can be conducted easily on a daily basis. Rural living carries with it a self-sufficiency that if not kept in check, can prevent those relationships from growing.

Think about the last time you received a letter and how it made you feel. Better yet, think about the last time you wrote one—the price of a stamp is well worth the priceless contents of a newsy letter from a friend or relation. With today's technology, email is another easy form of communication that connects family and friends. Sometimes it can be done instantly as with the messenger programs on some computers.

Phone calls are great, but the written word is cheaper.

It is also enduring. Old notes and letters give us tangible proof that someone was making the effort to stay in touch.

The proposal then is simple. Make a new habit. When the men are watching Monday Night Football, make some cookies, gather up paper and pen and write a letter to someone. Just don't forget to wipe the cookie crumbs off before sealing it in the envelope.

—Sue Jane

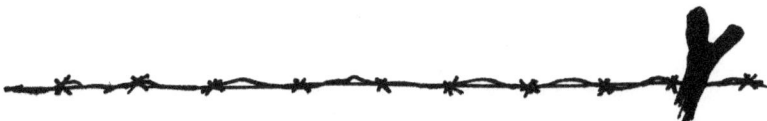

Capsule 23

Pass The Crackers and Keys, Please

*I*magine this—our vehicle is packed and Lola (the basset), my husband and I are about to make a getaway. We have a few extra days and are headed out of town. As we approach the outskirts of town, I turn toward the back of the "Jimmy" to get a snack from the usual supply of "road food" that we carry.

About that same time, it occurs to me to check on something important. "Do you have the keys?" I ask Jim Bob. His reply, "Sure," satisfies me that we will be able to get into the house at the vacation destination. Pleased with myself for asking before we reached the New Mexico line or some other point of no return, I settle into my seat to enjoy the ride and munch my crackers. A few minutes later, Mr. Jones (that's Jim Bob) gives me a strange look and says, "I thought you offered me some cheese—Were you just kidding?"

I had said, "Do you have the keys?" He heard, "Do you want some cheese?" That's not the first time that he has misunderstood something I said. But, it struck me as one of the funniest. While the result of hearing loss may prompt some funny situations, the loss of hearing is a serious matter. Missing parts of conversation is frustrating and can lead to incorrect conclusions, maybe even hard feelings. Trying to compensate for loss of hearing takes extra energy and reduces the pleasure one might find in social situations.

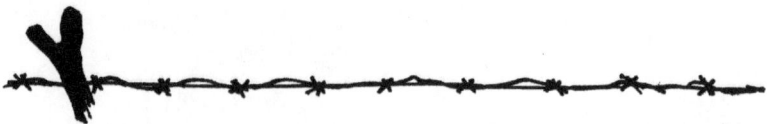

Several causes of hearing loss are not directly preventable. For example, acute infections may take their toll on the apparatus of sound transmission in an ear, some nerve tumors can cause deafness, and direct injury to the eardrum or other parts of the middle or inner ear can cause hearing loss. And some medications that are used to treat other illnesses may impair hearing, sometimes permanently. But, there is at least one type of hearing loss that is preventable. That is the loss associated with exposure to loud noises.

Hearing loss associated with noise is very similar to the loss that many experience with advanced age. That is, the tones (higher frequency) and loudness (softer volume) that are lost are the ones in the range of normal conversation. They are also the ones most like women's voices.

Are you thinking that just about everyone you know (particularly men) over 40 seems to have some of this type of hearing loss? It is possible that that could be the case, particularly if you know mostly people who are engaged in agriculture. Why? The reason is that, like my husband, many people who grew up on farms and ranches have been exposed to loud noise rather consistently. He spent many hours on the seat of a "poppin' Johnnie," the cabless tractor that lots of farm youths steered long before they could qualify to get a driver's license. The noise that is the culprit can be either short bursts of very loud sounds or lower volume sounds consistently over longer periods of time. Noise induced hearing loss is not something that happens only to men. We women are also subjected to "too loud, too much, too often." Think of the number of pieces of machinery on the farm or ranch that produce one or the other of those types of loud sounds. Irrigation motors, combines, cotton strippers, shredders, even shotguns and the .22 that you use to shoot varmints are on the list. Vacuum cleaners also create noxious noise.

Even with the improvement of farm machinery by the addition of cabs and air conditioning, the change in noise level is only a moderate improvement. Prevention of damage to the tiny nerve cells that transmit

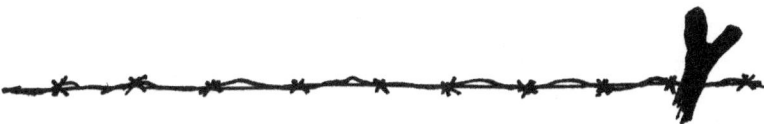

sound is, like many other types of prevention, a matter of being mindful. In the case of preventing hearing damage, the regular mindfulness relates to managing to avoid exposure to those loud noises.

One way to avoid the exposure is to get a job in town, I guess. And I wouldn't mind not running the vacuum. But, even away from agriculture, there is noise at every turn. A better answer is to use earplugs. Those little soft sponge ear protectors that airplane pilots use are a good choice. They are inexpensive and when they get dusty or are lost, they can be replaced. If these little helpers are in your pocket (or in your Ag-Pack) every day, then there is a good chance that you will remember to use them. Put them in at the first chance for consistent noise or for loud bursts of sound.

Why use them if you are already having hearing problems? Because there are degrees of hearing loss. You may be able to prevent further loss by reducing noise exposure. If you have an existing hearing problem, you should see a hearing specialist to have it evaluated. The source of the problem may be any one of the several types I mentioned above. If other types of hearing loss are present, why compound the problem by adding loud noise exposure?

One final word of advice. If you use the earplugs, don't forget to take them out when you go home or to town. If you keep them in, you could be in the same situation as my husband was that day—hoping for a snack and getting only crackers and a suggestion that now is the time to consider a hearing aid.

—Teddy

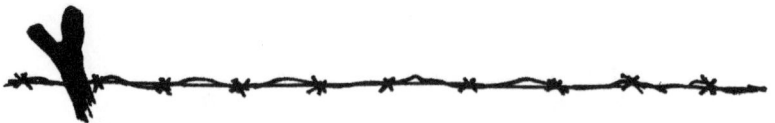

Capsule 24

A Sound I Prefer Not To Hear

*L*ate Fall has some special sounds here in West Texas. When a cold front arrives, there is the howl of the wind passing that legendary single strand of barbed wire between us and the North Pole. Occasional pops of shotgun fire and barking of retrievers indicate bird-hunting season. I particularly welcome the song of Sandhill Cranes. Their migratory "maps" include a long layover at the refuge near Muleshoe, about 30 miles from our place. Long before they descend and are visible, their sounds are a signal they have sighted fields with fallen grain to glean. Their cousins, the Whooping Cranes, arrive in this season on the Texas Gulf Coast at the Aransas Refuge. I am told that their whoop is distinctive. I would like to hear it.

But, there is another whoop I *do not* care to hear. That is the sound of pertussis—whooping cough. "Why worry," you might wonder, "there is a vaccination for that." True, there is an immunization for whooping cough and the incidence of the disease in the United States has declined dramatically with immunization. The problem is that while children who have been fully immunized are protected, infants who have not yet received the full initial series of four immunizations are not. Until the series is complete at around two years of age, they are not fully protected and those under six months are at the greatest risk, even if they have been started on the series.

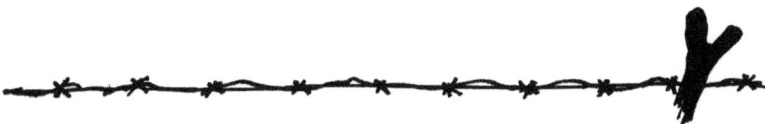

Here's the situation. Pertussis infection causes an illness that has three identifiable stages. Stage one is one to two weeks in length, following an incubation period of about seven to ten days. In this first stage, the person with "whooping cough" probably seems to have a common cold. There is a slow onset of runny nose, low grade fever and a mild occasional cough. It is during this early stage that the disease is most contagious. Like many other diseases, those who have it are passing it around without knowing it.

Rather than behaving like a common cold—improving and disappearing in a couple of weeks—pertussis moves into a second stage. The "paroxysmal cough" stage can last from one to six weeks. The person has rapid bursts of coughing—not just dainty throat clearing coughs—but hacking so violent it can break ribs. Because the coughing is rapid it leaves the person breathless. The following struggle to draw a breath results in a characteristic sound, a whoop. An average of 15 coughing attacks in a day is typical, increasing over the first week or two of this stage and then remaining at that level for another two to three weeks. A third stage is a convalescent period when, over another two to three weeks, the coughing spells decrease in number and finally stop.

Pertussis is treatable. Antibiotics can limit the infection and its severity. But, the problem is that the illness is most severe in infants because they can have the greatest number of complications and because the coughing leaves them weak. They may not have the strength to "whoop" and draw a breath. Instead, they suffer the results of limited oxygen. Their respiratory systems are not equipped for the violent demands of efforts to clear the airway in this disease. Further, because it begins like a common cold, whooping cough is often not diagnosed until the second stage and complications have begun. Complications can include pneumonia caused by other bacteria attacking the weakened lungs; neurologic problems caused by the reduced oxygen supply; middle ear infections; and dehydration. And results of the pressure created by

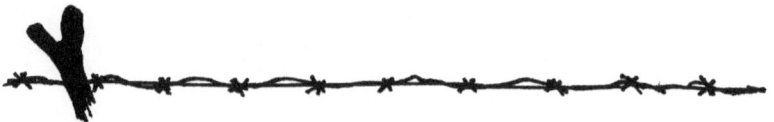

the coughing can include collapsed lung, nosebleed, and hernia.

Now here's the problem. Apparently, even though many who are now adults have been immunized, they may not have lifetime immunity and may contract pertussis. The Centers for Disease Control and Prevention reports research indicating that as many as 25% of adult illnesses presenting with cough persisting more that seven days may be attributable to pertussis. An adult typically has a less serious case of the infection and often can recover without treatment. But, they can transmit the whooping cough bacteria to infants.

What can you do? First, encourage anyone you know who has an infant to adhere to the schedule for immunizations. Second, if you have a cough that continues past seven days (particularly a violent cough) that is associated with a low-grade fever, see your health care provider. Ask if pertussis is a possibility. Third, if you have a cough, stay completely away from infants. As with so many respiratory illnesses, this one is spread by droplets sprayed by the cough.

—Teddy

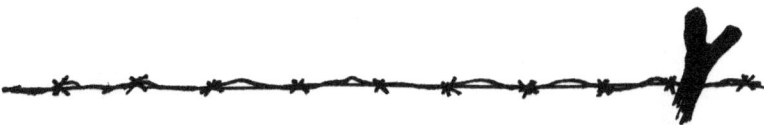

Capsule 25

A Good Understanding

My Othermama (doesn't everyone have a special name for their grandmothers?) came from Oklahoma to Texas in a covered wagon as a child. That trip, sometime around 1908, brought my mother's mother and all the large Head family. And they brought with them an interesting way of using words. She didn't speak a foreign language, but her "sayings" caught my imagination, as a child. Advice and descriptions became memorable when rendered in her special way. For example, one bit of advice that she conveyed was, "Be useful if you can't be ornamental." Certainly made me strive for usefulness, particularly since cosmetics never attracted me! A description she uttered, "That man surely has a good understanding," had nothing to do with a person's intelligence. She was talking about *big feet*. And feet are what I am talking about this time.

We hardly notice them—take them for granted, unless they begin to hurt or itch. But when they do become painful, dispositions sour and the search for relief consumes us. Why else is Dr. Scholl a household name? Some of the ills that affect our "understanding" are preventable. Like any prevention, it takes attention.

Corns and calluses are the easiest to deal with. Check your feet each time you bathe. Dry them well and look for any red or thickened spots. Those are pressure points. Friction and pressure encourage the

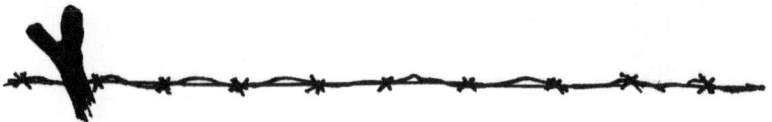

body to form protection. Protection gone awry is what becomes a callous or corn. Remove the thickened part by soaking and softening with hand lotion. Don't go trimming on the corn with your pocket-knife or a razorblade. One slip and you have a perfect spot for infection. You can use corn removal pads or you might need an abrasive pumice file to wear off a callous.

Then you have to search for the cause. Is it those new boots? Did a "sock wad" wear at you all day? What about high heels with a too small toe space? The best thing to do is to find the offending footwear and either work them over (I'm big on taking out insoles) or pass them on to someone else.

Did you ever notice that a pair of shoes that fit perfectly well for years suddenly hurts your feet? It could be because feet change. Look at a baby's fat little foot. Over the years, those fat pads tend to disappear. (I can see where mine went.) The result is less cushion and more opportunity for pressure points to develop. You can prevent some discomforts caused by "lean feet" by adding insoles for padding to any shoe or boot. You may need to consider changing shoe size too, because the longer we use our feet, the more likely they are to spread out. A wider shoe or one with a taller toe box may help.

Back to the idea of infection. If you are diabetic, it is especially easy to get an infection if you get a blister or have a small injury, like one self inflicted while corn paring. Because some diabetics have poor circulation and/or poor nerve conduction in the feet, infection can develop without awareness of pain. Big trouble. That's another reason for shoes that fit and for inspecting the feet each day.

The other common preventable foot problem is athlete's foot. You need never have been a jock to acquire this fungal infection. Women are not immune from it. It sits around just waiting for a chance to grow in a moist warm environment. Even children get it and when they wear their favorite pair of tennis shoes (the ones that cost a week's wage

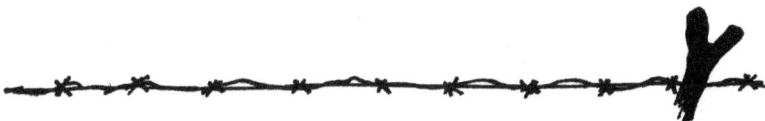

because they have lights in the heels) day after day, *tinea pedis* thrives. It is not just the tennis shoes—any shoe is like an oven if you have hot feet. Next thing you know, they are damp and so are your socks. There's the second ingredient—moisture. What can you do? If you already have athlete's foot, treat it. Some over-the-counter medicines that your pharmacist suggests can work for a minor case. Or, you may need a prescription for something stronger. It takes a long time to cure, so you have to be persistent about using the medicine.

To prevent or discourage reoccurrence, you need dry feet that stay cool. Socks that are made of fabric that "wicks" the moisture away from the feet are the best. Check labels or shop for them at a sporting goods store. Hikers have known about damp feet causing trouble for a long time, so the wicking socks are a favorite with them. Change socks during the day. Lunch and a socks change could only be improved on by making a shoe change at the same time!

And finally, you may have to ignore Merle Haggard if you want really cool, dry feet. In his song, "Okie From Muskogee," Merle sneered at wearing sandals, which he equated with hippie decadence. Merle's patriotism aside, I'll bet his feet never were dry—or cool. Sandals, with or without socks, are a really good choice for men, women and children any time you are "off duty" and not likely to drop something on your foot or to step in anything unfortunate.

Now that we have a "good understanding" on the subject, I believe I will go shopping for some shoes—something useful *and* ornamental. Maybe purple—sandals.

—Teddy

84

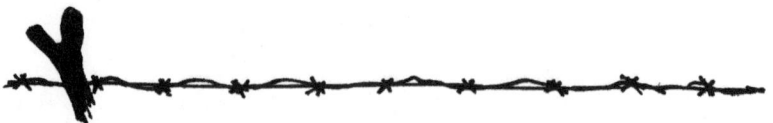

Capsule 26

What Momma Forgot to Tell Me

I have a lot in common with that guy Merle Haggard sings about in his song "Momma Tried." I'm not a convict, but I am a terrible cook. My mother was a great cook, she loved the kitchen, she modeled what I should have done, but this apple did fall far from the tree. When it comes to cooking or baking or preparing a meal, I simply do not like to.

Still, I was a practical person and knew that if marriage was in my future, these things would inevitably have to be done. So Momma gave me some excellent advice. She told me to keep it basic. Stick with what you know, what you like, what your husband likes, and don't worry about the fancy meals.

Being a right dutiful daughter, I took Momma's advice to heart and decided to get really good at a few things. And, if I was ever to be a hostess, I would prepare the things that I was most comfortable making. The only part of the meal equation that Momma forgot to tell me was that the foods really should complement each other.

I realize now that lasagna, fried potatoes, and homemade Butterfinger ice cream are not exactly complements. But the criteria fit: I loved them, I enjoyed preparing them, and I was good at it.

Even my friends got used to the combination. In fact, it became a draw to get people to drive the 30 miles out in the country to visit us just to eat this meal. I think my family was skeptical, but soon my

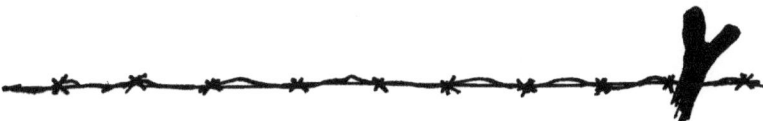

reputation flourished. I was fixing lasagna for my husband's boss, for my kids' friends, for my neighbors. Fried potatoes—a great recipe my mother-in-law had given me—had to be served, too, because they just seemed to go with the lasagna.

In later years, when I got really good in the kitchen, I added a fruit salad and some French bread, but they were merely tokens.

The grand finale was, of course, the homemade Butterfinger ice cream. We soon outgrew the four-quart container and moved up the tall six-quart cylinder. The taste was just as good because I added another can of condensed milk, one more cup of sugar, three more eggs, but no more Mexican vanilla because I was afraid of exceeding the .08 BAC. Three more Butterfingers were thrown in for added flavor. Maybe four. I lose count.

Maybe I misinterpreted some of Momma's advice, but the end result has proven successful. My family and friends can count on me for one decent meal. Below are the recipes for success as I have discovered through the years, and I gladly share them with you in hopes that this Southern Fried Italian French cuisine will delight your guests for years to come.

Thanks, Mom. I owe it all to you—including the 25 pounds I've put on since I got married.

UNINSPIRED WOMAN-IN-THE-KITCHEN LASAGNA

    1 box of oven-ready lasagna noodles
    salt, pepper, oregano to taste
    2 to 3 lbs. ground meat (depending on your taste)
    1 pkg. Swiss cheese slices
    8 oz. can of tomato sauce
    1 pkg. Mozzarella cheese
    1 large container of cottage cheese

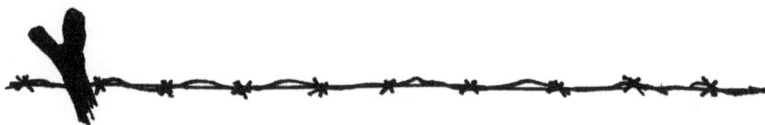

Brown meat. Drain and rinse (personal preference). Season. Add tomato sauce. Stir around for awhile. In a 9 x 12 dish (or whatever that rectangular size pan is), place a layer of noodles on the bottom, top with a layer of cottage cheese, a layer of Swiss cheese, a layer of Mozzarella cheese, and then top that with the meat sauce. Repeat the layer.

Bake at 350 for 45 minutes till bubbly. Let stand for about 5 minutes before serving.

MOTHER-IN-LAW FRIED POTATOES*

4-5 large potatoes	½ cup flour
dash of sugar	salt and pepper
cooking oil	cast iron skillet/lid

Heat cooking oil in skillet. Peel potatoes and slice like you were making French fries. Wash and rinse potatoes after peeling.

Put in large bowl, salt and pepper to taste, and then sprinkle about ½ cup flour over the potatoes along with one tsp. of sugar. Toss and mix well.

Put potatoes in the skillet, cover, and fry on medium temp. Keep the lid on and turn every ten minutes or so. You want the potatoes to get soft. Once they do, drain off most but not all of the oil. Turn up the heat, re-cover, and fry until crusty brown. Turn every minute or so. Completely drain oil, add a little more salt and pepper to taste, keep covered until ready to serve.

* From my ex-mother-in-law Patsy Mayes who learned how to make potatoes like this from her mother-in-law, Delma Mayes back in Wichita Falls, Texas, in the 1950s. Thanks, Pat!

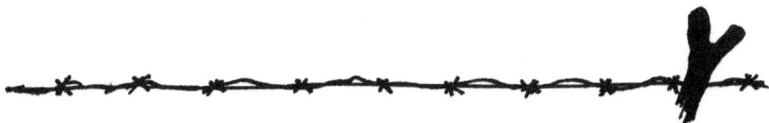

GRAND FINALE: HOMEMADE BUTTERFINGER ICE CREAM

This recipe is for a six-quart freezer (four-quart measurements in parentheses).

9 eggs (6)	5 large Butterfingers (6 medium)
2 tsp. Mexican vanilla (1)	3 ½ cups sugar (2)

1 ½ cans sweetened condensed milk (1)

2% milk about ½ gallon

1 box rock salt, plenty of ice, and a good ice cream freezer

I do not cook my eggs because my cousin Pierce, a chef, told me I did not have to. So there. But I do have to beat them. After the eggs are going on medium speed in the mixer, add the sweetened condensed milk and mix for five minutes. Add the sugar and mix for five more. Put the Butterfingers in a large freezer bag (a little more durable) and beat them with something like a hammer or a meat cleaver. Pour them into the bowl and let that mix well for 2 or 3 minutes. Add vanilla. Pour into freezer container. Add 2% milk to the fill line on the freezer. Freeze. After the motor stops, drain off the salt water, take out the dash, cover with plastic wrap and replace the lid, and then add ice and salt again to the top of the freezer. Pack with an old towel and let that set for 20 minutes.

—Sue Jane

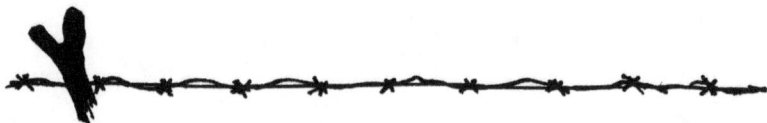

Capsule 27

Something Fishy

Do you remember cod liver oil? I mean, did you ever really have to hold your nose and swallow it because your grandmother said you needed it? I don't (and didn't) but "way back then" cod liver oil was thought to have health benefits, particularly for children with poor diets. We know now that one of the reasons for the oil's benefit is its high content of Vitamins A and D.

Research continues on the health effects of elements of diet and dietary supplements (including cod liver oil). As findings of various studies become available, scientific groups interested in providing guidance to health care providers and the general public evaluate the studies. One group that performs this service is the American Heart Association (AHA). The scientific panels of the AHA look at the result of studies *and* at the quality of the research (design, number of subjects, possible confounding factors). Using this review method, they develop statements related to their area of concern. Such official statements of recognized organizations are far more reliable then the sensational reports of single research studies in the popular media. In short, there's nothing "fishy" about the recommendation that the AHA publishes, based on this careful approach. (www.americanheart.org)

However, the subject of one of their statements published in late 2002, "Fish Consumption, Fish Oil, Omega-3 Fatty Acids and Cardio-

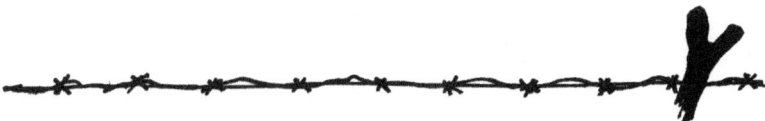

vascular Disease" is (fishy, I mean). Twenty-two pages, with 119 references, it echoes those in their 1996 statement on the same subject. Summary: EAT FISH.

At the risk of offense to hog farmers, poultry raisers, cattle ranchers, and emu breeders, I am convinced that adding some fish to our diets can be beneficial. Besides, isn't fish farming an agricultural enterprise?

The beneficial element in the fish is omega-3 fatty acids. Fish are the most direct dietary source. The alpha-lineoleic acid in some plant oil sources is partially converted to omega-3, and can be of benefit as well.

So, you ask, how much fish are we talking about? As with many questions, the correct answer is "it depends." Fatty fish have the most omega-3 fatty acids in them, so less of that type of fish is needed. Salmon, herring, sardines, and fresh tuna are among the highest. But, even canned white tuna can be a beneficial source as can trout. In general, the cold water fish are the ones with the highest content. The recommendation for healthy people is two servings per week of about three ounces each. That assumes that you attempt to use some of the higher content fish as part of that ration. That also means you can trade in just one bologna sandwich or burrito for a big fat tuna sandwich, preferably on whole grain bread, and you're halfway there. And any is better than none.

Unfortunately for those of us who like those crunchy fried bits that a fast food fish restaurant tempts us with, the benefits of fish prepared by the fast-food-fried methods are cancelled out by the transfats used in deep-frying. So, broiled is best. If you are the family grocery shopper, you will notice that some stores are now carrying filets, both fresh and frozen, that are cut in the handy three-ounce size.

After adding that one other fish meal each week, try using canola, walnut, soybean, or olive oil in food preparation as salad dressing,

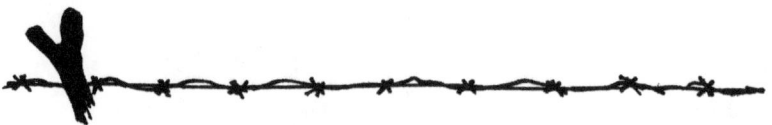

margarine, or for frying or basting. That adds the plant-based source of some omega-3.

The only warnings about increasing fish consumption have to do with possible mercury contamination of fish, particularly in sport-caught fish and fresh tuna. So, only a portion of the fish consumed should come from these. Pregnant women and children should use other sources.

People with known heart disease or elevated triglyceride levels can benefit from even higher intake of omega-3 fatty acids. Consult your health care provider for guidance on diet and/or supplements if you have either of those diagnoses. By the way, one of the least expensive supplements supplying omega-3 fatty acids is—you guessed it, cod liver oil.

—Teddy

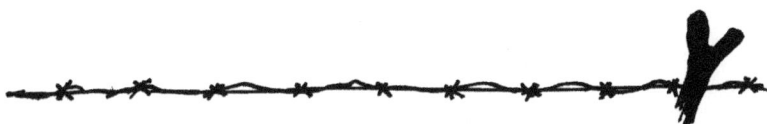

Capsule 28

Being Compliant Is Not Easy, Maybe Not Natural

"*B*ut why?" Those may have been the earliest words I learned, right after Mama, I mean. Although the lessons of childhood and much of my education discouraged me from always uttering them, they were always there. I wondered *why* I should enjoy running the footraces my third grade teacher instigated at recess. "*Why?*" I wrote on my plane geometry notes when we were told that certain rules were "givens." I could fill this page with occasions when "but why?" preceded any act of compliance on my part.

As a health care provider, I have found myself understanding the patients who are labeled by my colleagues as "non-compliant." Those are the patients who don't do what we ask (or tell) them to do. Or if they do follow instructions, they find ways to change them to suit themselves. Some will choose to take a medication only as long as the most distressing symptoms are present, stopping as soon as they feel a little better. Others nod dutifully that they understand the need to lose weight and then never increase their exercise or decrease their food intake. There are countless examples of choices that patients make that earn them the "non-compliant" title.

But, I understand. I understand for two reasons. First, it is not always easy to comply with health related advice or instructions. Reasons include:

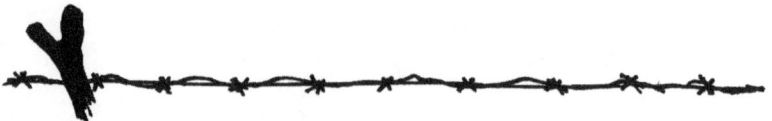

- the instructions are complicated, unclear
- inconvenient changes in routine or habit are required
- doing something unpleasant or distasteful is required

A recent experience set me thinking about compliance. Actually, I was thinking about non-compliance, because I was flirting, once again, with being that; with letting "but why?" rule my actions. Annual physical exam just completed, I was about to thank my doctor and leave when she handed me an envelope. "You know what this is, a stool specimen kit for colorectal cancer screening. Be sure you do it and mail it back. Now don't forget."

I didn't ask, "But why?" I knew the answer for this one. Colorectal cancer is the second leading cancer killer each year in the United States. Annual screening such as this test can reduce colorectal cancer deaths by as much as 50% because with early detection, a 90% cure rate is possible. All men and women over age 50 should have this test, annually. An additional test, sigmoidoscopy, is recommended every 5 years after age 50.

It was when I got home and opened the envelope that I began to consider non-compliance. Instructions filled a full page in small print. They included among other thing, avoiding all red meat for three days prior to and during the three days of the test; avoiding vitamin C in excess of 250 mg./day from citrus juice or fruits; and removing toilet bowl cleaner from the toilet tank and flushing twice before "proceeding," as they put it so delicately. In addition to the instructions, there were three cardboard packets, each with two slots for specimens and DO NOT OPEN printed on the back flap. These were accompanied by a special mailing envelope suitable for biohazardous material, three collection tissues (I won't go into the instructions for *their* use) and three wooden sticks too small to eat ice cream from. Referring again to the

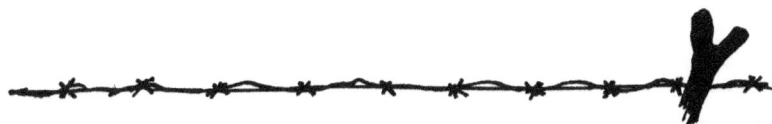

instructions, I noted that I was not to flush those sticks.

Even though I knew why I should do the test and wanted to comply, that package was daunting. It fits all three of the usual reasons for non-compliance that I mentioned before: complicated, inconvenient, distasteful.

And then there's the second reason I understand those who have trouble complying. There are some of us for whom it is JUST NOT NATURAL TO COMPLY, at least not until we ask, "But why?"

There I was, wavering, on the brink between my nature and good sense. Plane geometry came to my rescue. I remembered that for the first two six-weeks of the 10th grade, I had barely made a C in the course. The third six-weeks was when I decided that I would just accept the "givens." My grade shot up to an A.

After I performed the necessary rituals to complete the colorectal screening test and mailed it away, I was at peace. I knew that, as in plane geometry, I had complied when the evidence told me it was in my best interest.

But, I had also reserved the right to exercise my basic nature to always ask, "But why?" If you and I have that trait in common, I hope you will think of this story the next time you receive advice from your health care provider.

—Teddy

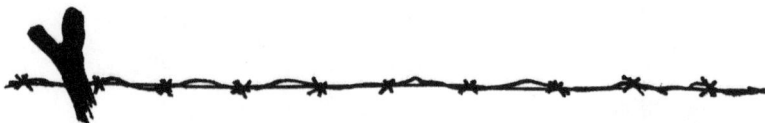

Capsule 29

They've Got My Number

I was thinking about my Social Security number. Since I began work at Berry's Drug in Iowa Park, Texas, at the age of 13, that number has been mine. I understand that it identifies me with an account held by the government from which someday a pension is to be paid to me. While some money may or may not materialize when the time comes, the number has identified me in lots of situations and it is mine, whether I like it or not. Unless I go into a Witness Protection Program, it is not going to change.

But, there are some numbers that we can change. One from a long list of potentially changeable numbers is my cholesterol. If you have visited a health screening, you may have "gotten your number" for cholesterol. That screening, along with blood pressure and blood glucose, is offered at such events because it is an important clue to risk of heart disease.

The single number (total cholesterol) that you receive in such a screening is useful in that, if it is elevated (over 200), it suggests a need to take health-promoting action. For those with total cholesterol over 240 (or over 200 if there are other risk factors of heart disease such as smoking, family history, diabetes or obesity) additional numbers are important, also. Those are the numbers from a lipoprotein analysis. That identifies the high-density "good" cholesterol and the low-density "bad"

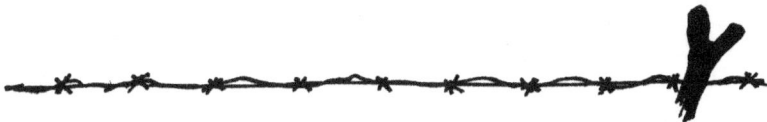

cholesterol portions of the total. This helps your health care provider determine what actions are needed.

Understanding how the fats in the blood operate is a bit like understanding what happens with the money that goes to Social Security in care of that unchangeable number I was issued. Both are pretty complicated. I can do a better job of explaining something about the fats than explaining anything about government. But, be warned, continuing research changes what is known. As more is discovered about the relationship of various fat components to disease, recommendations change. And, it is important to keep in mind that cholesterol is just one factor that is known to relate to cardiovascular disease.

Back to the explanation. Cholesterol is a fat molecule that is both manufactured by the body and is taken into the body through the diet. Even if dietary intake of fats is entirely absent, the body must manufacture some due to cholesterol's necessary role in creating cell membranes, reproductive and steroid hormones and bile acids. Cholesterol is transported in the blood attached to protein molecules as lipoproteins. About 75% of the cholesterol is bound to Low-Density Lipoproteins (LDL) and 25% to High-Density Lipoproteins (HDL). Therefore, HDL + LDL = Total Cholesterol. Because LDL is the one associated with cholesterol that "settles out" and forms plaques in the blood vessels, the desirable situation is for the LDL to be low and the HDL to be high, as portions of the total cholesterol. Because of the 75/25 ratio of LDL to HDL, the total needs to be relatively low (less than 200) to assure that the LDL stays in acceptable limits.

Several factors can affect a person's cholesterol. They include: gender—women usually have lower cholesterol until after menopause; exercise—active exercise can lower cholesterol; diet—a high fat diet raises cholesterol; medications—several drugs, including beta blockers, oral contraceptives, and thiazide diuretics can increase cholesterol; genetic differences—some people are genetically "programmed" to metabolize

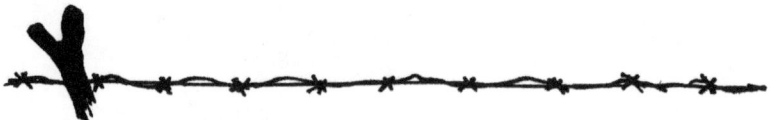

fats better or more poorly than others; smoking—increases cholesterol; stress—there it is again!

Can a person alter their cholesterol and thereby their cardiac risks without medication? Looking at those factors that elevate cholesterol, it's clear that many of them are things we can affect. In fact, the Expert Panel on Detection, Evaluation and Treatment of High Blood Cholesterol in Adults indicate that a six-month trial of changes in modifiable factors should precede a decision to use medication for most patients without other major risk factors. Alter what? Exercise and diet for starters. We cannot change our genetic patterns, but we can change behavior. Information surrounds us—about lower fat diets, about exercise for folks of any age and ability—it is a matter of choosing to use it.

I like that. I *like* the idea that if my cholesterol shoots up, I can take the opportunity to use some good sense, some effort and a bit of self-control to change the number. Okay, call me goofy, it's just sort of pleasing to know that, especially since I can't change my Social Security number.

—Teddy

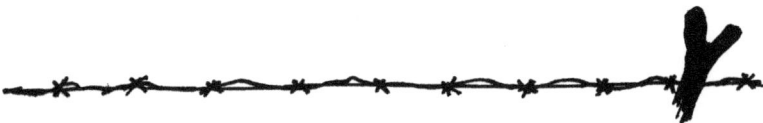

Capsule 30

Get In Line For Another Number

You may recall I've mentioned important numbers, cholesterol and Social Security. Now, I am offering another number that you need to know. Blood glucose is a figure that can be checked easily with the blood from just a finger-stick. Of course, it can also be measured as a part of a panel of tests performed on whole blood drawn from a vein. But, it's a fact that many of us avoid stopping in at the local health care provider when we have no symptoms. The reasoning goes something like this, "I'm feeling okay and if I go in there they will keep looking until they find something wrong." I will leave trying to change your mind about that for another day. For now, I will just suggest that the next time a free or low cost glucose screening is offered, you line up and "get a number."

The glucose test can be done fasting or random. If you haven't had anything but water for 8-12 hours, the fasting level would be used as index of normal. A normal fasting glucose is less than 100 mg/dl. Above 126 mg/dl is a diabetic level and between 101 and 125 is called pre-diabetes or impaired fasting glucose. For a random test (anything other than fasting), up to 200 mg/dl is normal. But, if it has been more than 2 hours since eating, the number should be lower than 140 mg/dl to be considered normal and not pre-diabetic. That's because it should

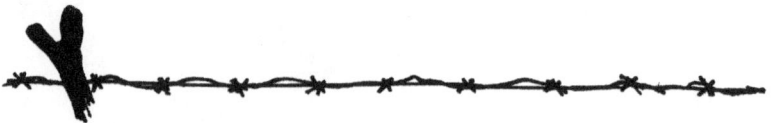

be heading back toward the fasting level if your body is handling properly the glucose that is extracted from your food.

If the screening shows the glucose to be above normal, that's a signal to visit your health care provider, pronto. The reason for concern is that high blood glucose usually indicates diabetes, either Type 1 or Type 2. I say usually because there are a few other conditions that can prompt an elevated blood glucose. But the most common is diabetes.

Most of us have a friend or relative with diabetes. Increasing awareness and better diagnostic methods have helped identify more cases, earlier than in the past. So, it is fairly well known that diabetes mellitus (the proper name) is the condition in which there is either a lack of insulin produced by the pancreas and/or malfunction in the use of glucose and insulin at the level of the cells in the body. Glucose is necessary for cell function. Insulin is required to help the glucose move across the cell membrane in the cell. So, if there is insufficient insulin, the glucose is not used by the cells. Or, if there is a malfunction at the cellular level, even if the insulin is there, there is a resistance to its ability to move the glucose into the cell where it can be utilized.

When the lack of insulin is the main problem, that is called Type 1 Diabetes Mellitus. Type 2 is diagnosed when the cellular resistance is the main difficulty, although there may also be decline in or absence of production of insulin. Generally, Type 2 develops in people past the age of 30, while Type 1 is more often identified in younger people. Type 1 accounts for about 10% of cases and Type 2, 90%. In either case, the result is that glucose is extracted from the digestion of food, but is not used efficiently. The excess floats in the bloodstream doing damage. It damages the small blood vessels in the eyes, the kidneys, and in the entire circulatory system as well as the peripheral nerves.

Type 2 Diabetes tends to develop more gradually and while there is still much that's not known about why people develop diabetes of

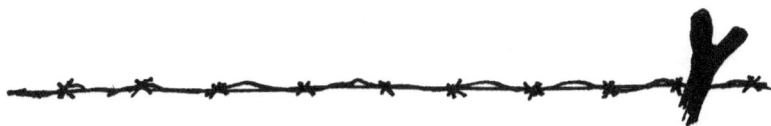

either type, some risk factors are known. For example, for Type 2, obesity and lack of exercise are two big ones. Genetics also plays a role because the incidence of diabetes is higher for those with a first degree relative with diabetes and for Native Americans, Hispanics, African Americans and Asians.

Since we do not get to choose our parents, the main risk factors we can affect are the weight and exercise. Yes, that again! I do mention those factors often for some reason or other.

Diabetes is not like a cold—it won't go away if you just get some rest. Rather, diabetes is sneaky. It can begin to cause eye and kidney damage while a person is busy ignoring the early symptoms (extreme thirst, increased urination, fatigue).

The good news is that good treatment and self-care can reduce the incidence of damage and can make the disease far more manageable that was the case in the past. Early diagnosis is the key. So, the next time you see a glucose screening, line up—get your number.

—Teddy

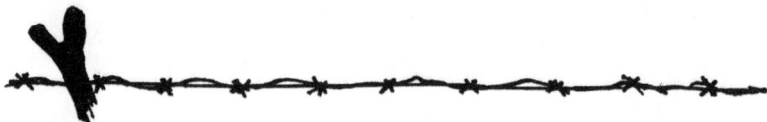

Capsule 31

Sticks And Stones

Sticks and stones may break my bones. So begins the little ditty from childhood. We can all complete the verse. But, here's an alternate verse that can serve as a useful reminder. "Sticks and stones may break my bones, but osteoporosis is a far more likely source of fracture." Okay, so it doesn't rhyme!

Osteoporosis exists when the strength of the bones of the skeleton is reduced and the bones are at increased risk of fracture. Bone strength can be affected by: 1) the quality of the bone structure created during childhood and adolescence, and 2) the extent of loss of bone as a person ages. Women are more likely than men to be affected by osteoporosis and among women, small-boned Caucasian women and Asian women have the greatest likelihood of developing the problem. However, lower risk for men does not mean that a man has no reason to be concerned. Rather, if the man lives to a "ripe old age" his chances of developing osteoporosis rise with age. That is because men typically develop a larger, heavier skeleton than women during their growth years (before age 20). So, if bone loss begins in a male, it becomes a problem later for the person who started with the larger frame.

If being a bit "light in the bones" doesn't strike you as much of a problem, consider this. Most hip and vertebral fractures are prompted by osteoporosis. It is not a fall alone that causes the fracture. It only

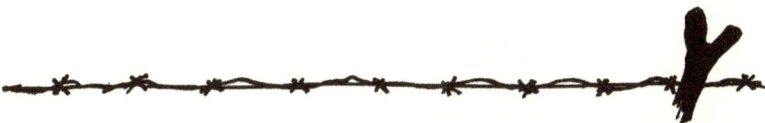

contributes and causes a break when the bones are weak.

The advertising on television and in print media for medication to treat osteoporosis and for bone mineral density testing to diagnosis it may have raised awareness about the need to TREAT osteoporosis. But, at least as important, and far less expensive, as treatment is prevention.

Prevention can focus on: 1) developing a strong skeleton during the growing years, and 2) preventing excessive bone loss as a person ages. Skeletal growth of a child is affected by genetics, but the best genetically determined potential can only be reached with adequate nutrition. (I know I am not telling farmers and ranchers anything new. Nutritional quantity and quality are essential for both crops and animals to reach their greatest potential also.)

With regard to bone, calcium and vitamin D are major requirements. Dairy products and sunshine are the handiest sources for these respectively. Weight-bearing exercise also strengthens bones. For the first few months of life, breastfeeding or a good formula feeding pretty much takes care of everything until about six months of age. But, after that, particularly at the teen years, the story changes. A report from the National Institutes of Health estimates that only 25% of boys and 10% of girls in the U.S., ages 9–17, meet daily calcium intake recommendations. For that matter, only about 50–60% of older adults meet the recommendations for their age.

Dietary intake of calcium is a desirable way for both adults and children to get the recommended amounts of calcium and other nutrients. For people who do not eat dairy products, dark green leafy vegetables and sardines also supply calcium. Some cereals and breakfast bars are fortified with calcium also. An eight-ounce glass of milk or serving of yogurt contains about 300 mg. of calcium. The chart below shows the recommended amount of calcium at various ages. If a person is not getting that amount during the growth years, the skeleton does not develop full size and strength. If the intake is inadequate in adult years,

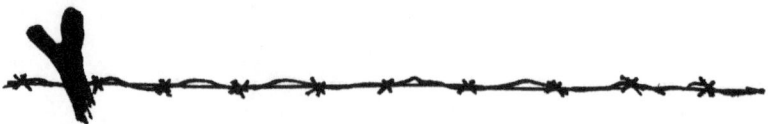

bone loss can occur. This is because bone, a living tissue, is constantly being reformed. When there is not enough available calcium, a net loss of bone can result from the reforming process.

Recommended Calcium Intake in Milligrams/Day

Age	Mg./day
Birth-6 months	210
6 months – 1 year	270
1.1 year – 3.99 years	500
4 years – 8.99 years	800
9 years – 13.99 years	1300
14 years – 18.99 years	1300
19 years – 30.99 years	1000
31 years – 50.99 years	1000
51 years – 70 years	1200
Older than 70 years	1200

In the adult years, some factors in addition to calcium intake can increase bone loss. These include: 1) estrogen reduction in postmenopausal women, 2) excessive alcohol intake, 3) cigarette smoking, 4) limited weight bearing exercise, and 5) medications prescribed for other illness which may have a side effect of altering the bone reforming process in some way.

The prevention message? Consume enough calcium or supplement as needed, exercise regularly, reduce alcohol consumption if excessive, stop smoking, and check with your health care provider about the desirability of other medications if you are past menopause. If you take medication for a chronic illness, check also about any effect that the drugs might have on bone strength.

—Teddy

Capsule 32

Another Trip to Bountiful

*A*unt Eula flew to Texas last summer from Yakima, Washington, for our McCleskey family reunion. Nearing 87 and in poor health, this was probably her last trip to her native state, a place she left in the post-World War II days of 1946.

Her husband had been a glider pilot during the war, and Uncle Hughy was anxious to take his bride of two years back to his home in Yakima. But, he promised her when they married that she could make yearly trips back to Fisher County to see her mother, my grandmother.

He kept that promise, partly with Aunt Eula's help, as she continued to teach second grade even after her two children were born.

When my grandmother died in 1955, the yearly trips ended but Aunt Eula still visited often because the farm in Texas was and would always remain home.

On Sunday morning of the reunion, my cousins and brothers and sisters and our children left Lubbock for the two-hour trip to the farm, some 11 miles northeast of the little town of Rotan, Texas. Aunt Eula became ill on the way down, so when we arrived in Rotan it was decided to move her to my car since it had tinted windows, which would help keep her a little cooler.

The round-trip to the farm and back from Rotan—22 miles—was

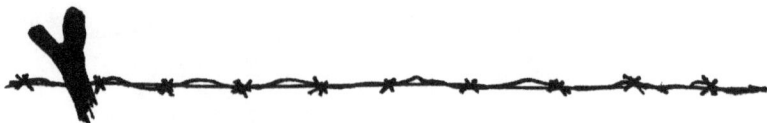

brief, but in that short time I saw and heard a precious reflection of her memories from days long gone.

Hunched over by osteoporosis, Aunt Eula barely could see over the dash of my small car, but she was all eyes as she strained to look at the cotton fields and mesquites on this dry piece of Texas.

The red soil south of the Double Mountains covered my car, as we were the last in a five-car caravan on the dusty roads. Along the way I heard her tell about where the Tommy Helms family lived and where her cousin Robert had stayed. The old Hodo place was gone as were many of the terraces that had eroded since her last visit in 1990. As we neared the farm, each turn, each dwelling, brought a recollection to her mind. Telling me those stories seemed to be to be a way of confirming the place in her heart that this first home held.

She showed me where her best friend, Mary Martin, had lived. Mary and Aunt Eula both left their farm homes to go on to college in Abilene in 1933—Mary to Hardin-Simmons University and Aunt Eula to Abilene Christian College. Even there in Abilene, she said, they would walk across open fields to visit, just as they had done as girls back home in Fisher County. The final turn brought us to the homestead where Aunt Eula had lived with my grandparents from her birth in 1916, along with the four siblings who followed.

Certainly it was too hot and she was too feeble to allow for one last walk, but we found a pear tree for shade down in the orchard. Here we set up the lawn chair, nestled between some cotton rows. What she wouldn't have given for that luxury 75 years earlier!

Sitting quietly in this spot, Aunt Eula recalled the evenings when her father had taught her, the eldest of five, to drive in those fields. These lessons came, ironically, just months before he died after cleaning out a well on the family property.

My cousin Linda collected some of the red soil for her mother to

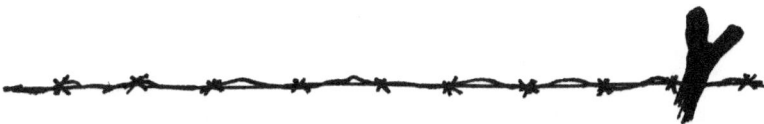

put in a plastic bag to take back to Washington. At one time, it had been "just dirt" to me and still was just dirt to the younger ones this day who were throwing a few clods, kicking up a little dust.

Even in the midst of the playing around, though, the second and third generation McCleskeys seemed to know they were witnessing a rite of passage. It is easy to take such moments for granted, to be oblivious, but on this Sunday morning it appeared we all were aware of the significance. Aunt Eula would fly home Tuesday, and we would not see her in Texas again.

The other thing that became clear that Sunday is that home is many places.

Sentimentally, Aunt Eula's home has remained Texas; physically it became Washington. That's where she lived most of her life, had her children, and taught school for over 30 years. It's where she'll be buried beside Uncle Hughy someday. But neither Texas nor Washington can claim her for much longer.

"Home is where we're going," according to writer Louis L'Amour.

Beyond the obvious eternal reward she's going to have, Aunt Eula is already much at home in other important places.

Those places are, in the words of poet Elizabeth Barret Browning, quite nearby, "...tell thy soul their roots are left in mine."

Not many young people today have such roots, and if they do, they neglect—as do many adults—to nurture them. Family connections lose their depth and become nothing but names in a baby book.

The brief 22-mile round trip to the farm and back to Rotan just watered those roots for my family as we *saw*, not just listened to, Aunt Eula's memories.

Aunt Eula gave us all something at Sunday's farm visit that will be forever with us—a look back so that we can appreciate what lies ahead. That's what roots do—provide strength below so that growth can take place on the surface.

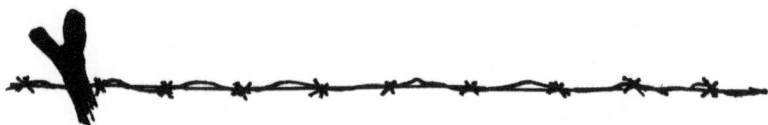

Along with the farm, that's a lesson this family hopes to hold on to for generations to come.

—Sue Jane

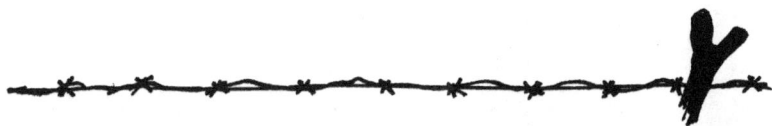

Capsule 33

Show Me...

*I*f there's anything more common than cell phones these days, it is people talking about how much stress they have. You'll even hear little kids saying, "I'm so stressed out about my music recital." Adults can be heard explaining their own cranky behavior. "I guess it is just the stress from the uncertainty about the Farm Program." No one seems to blame anything good on stress and everyone can list several things to blame on it.

Well, I am here to say something good about stress. Without some stress, life would be mighty dull. What? A health care provider thinking kindly of stress? If that seems a little odd, I will try to explain.

Stress is the response of an organism to any potentially damaging stimulus. Notice I said organism. Stress affects all beings—animals, plants, and even amoebas. The man who used the word stress to describe this response first was Dr. Hans Selye. Back in the 1950s and 60s, he did the research that brought stress in humans to public attention. To understand stress, it is important to know how he described it.

First, stress is the *response* we have to what happens, not what happens. The things that cause stress are—well, almost anything. They are called stressors. Extremes of temperature, physical danger, cattle prods, crowding, isolation, too much food, too little food, disease organisms, cell phones, excess work, extreme exertion, emotional loss

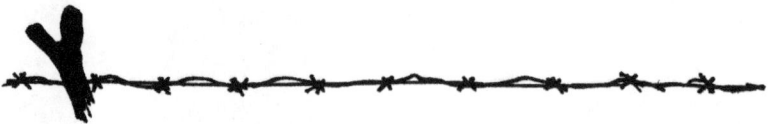

or threat of loss. You name it, it can cause stress if it poses a threat—actual or imagined to any part of us—body, mind or spirit.

When a stressor affects us, a series of reactions occur. Those reactions were what Dr. Selye first called the General Adaptation Syndrome, what we now call stress. If the organism is healthy, it reacts with alarm, sending the blood pressure up, focusing our attention, increasing alertness, reducing blood flow to the stomach and sending more to the muscles, pumping out adrenaline and other stress hormones, increasing stomach acid, boosting the immune system and in general getting us ready to "fight back." If the stressor is dealt with effectively by these defenses, the person has adapted. That adaptation used some energy. But, overall, it's a success for the human organism. So what's the problem? The problems caused by stress occur when the organism "isn't up to it" because of repeated stress which has used up all its energy for adaptation. This is when *distress* is happening. That is when the trouble starts.

How much is too much? I mentioned that stress can be enjoyable, giving a feeling of being able and up to challenges. That's how I feel when I manage to plow all day without going in the ditch. Yes, the plowing assignment is a stressor to me, but the stress makes me alert. Now, you've probably driven a tractor most of your life, so it isn't a stressor to you. There's the point—stress is an individual thing. What prompts my stress is not entirely the same as yours.

The same is true for how much stress is too much. It differs for each one of us from day to day and differs from person to person. Each of us has a point each day where stress can become distress.

Managing stress means keeping it at the level where it is not *distress*, but is *eustress*-just the right amount to feel alive and alert. Managing stress well means we have to recognize the signs that it is above that enjoyable level. Since we each are unique, our signals are individual as well. For some of us, distress is first signaled by a headache.

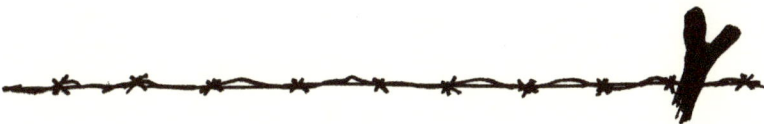

For others, a backache is the clue. Nausea or stomach pain or other gastrointestinal upsets are common signs. Another person may feel something more subtle, not pain, but agitation or irritability. Each of these is the result of an exaggeration of some aspect of the "ready to fight" reactions of the stress response. Changes in blood flow, muscle tension, increased gastric acid, hyperalertness are all initially useful. When they are prolonged or exaggerated, they become signals of distress. They should not be ignored with, "Oh, it's only stress." Rather, they should prompt us to take action to manage the stress.

Overall, there are three general ways to manage stress. One is to do something directly to eliminate the stressor. A second is to improve the general condition of the "organism" to make us better able to adapt, and the third is to change how we respond to the stressor, particularly how we think about it.

If that sounds to you like a tall order, you're right. If managing stress were not a chore, people who make lots of money selling self-help books and medicines and doing counseling would be out of work. Stress management can be learned. But, knowing about it is not enough. It takes practice. Think of it as a kind of maintenance chore like keeping the fences mended or the motors lubricated.

Until you have more skill with those tactics, aim to manage stress effectively, not avoid it entirely. Enjoy the excitement of *eustress*. Remember this: "Show me a person without stress and I will show you someone who is not really alive."

—Teddy

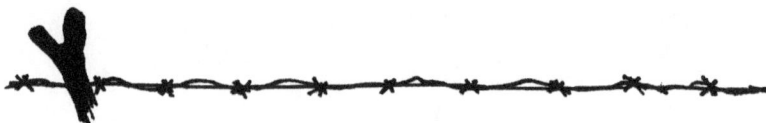

Capsule 34

Talking To Yourself...And Other Healthy Activities

"*J*ust relax," I was talking to myself again. "Whoa'" you're thinking, "do I want to take advice about stress management from a woman who talks to herself?" That's a legitimate question. We often think of talking to oneself as a sign of a rather loose attachment to reality. But, I think I can convince you that talking to ourselves can be healthy if you will read on.

Stress is a natural part of life. Some stress is necessary and beneficial but when it becomes *distress*, we need to learn methods to manage it. So, managing stress is what this is all about—including the part about talking to ourselves.

Stress is the response we have when we encounter anything that is a stressor and provokes a defensive response. The ways that we can manage stress can be put in three categories. Those are: 1) put the organism (that's you) in the best possible condition to respond, 2) remove the stressor or remove yourself from the stressor, and 3) change how you think about the stressor. Let's focus on that first category.

Put the Organism in the Best Possible Condition. Staying generally healthy is one of the best methods to put a person in the best possible condition. "That's pretty obvious. Say something useful," I am telling myself. Simple as that sounds, it is an important point. A person who is tired from lack of sleep, whose muscles are not well conditioned, whose

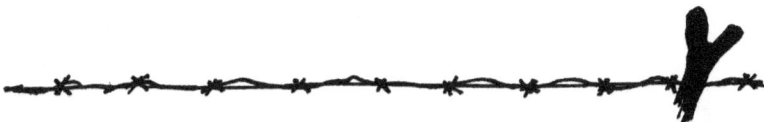

blood sugar is low from lack of regular food intake, or who is weakened by even a relatively minor infection such as a cold will experience distress more readily than one who is in the "best possible condition." That's why the really basic good health habits are important in being prepared to deal with stress.

Practicing specific relaxation methods can also put the organism in good condition. There are several techniques for creating the relaxation response. One of those is relaxation breathing.

Here's how. Breathe in while mentally counting to eight-letting the air reach all the way down to the bottom of the lungs. (Notice how seldom breath goes that deep!) Then exhale just as slowly, ending on the count of eight.

When you have breathed that way for five minutes, you will have the rhythm and not need to count. For the second five minutes, instead of counting, think as you inhale "breathe in a deep cleansing breath." As you exhale, think "let out every bit of the stress." Ten minutes of that routine twice a day will improve your lung capacity *and* give you a way to respond when you feel tension and stress begin to build. Then, the next time a steer goes through the electric fence and leads 30 of his friends along, before you do anything else, you do a couple of minutes of relaxation breathing. You will be surprised how much better you will manage. And, as you notice, talking to yourself, at least mentally, makes perfect sense in this exercise.

Another method for relaxation is imagery. This may take a little more practice than the relaxation breathing because it requires that you close your eyes (which means that you shouldn't do this while driving your pickup). It has been proven valuable as a way of causing a relaxation response, and in fact, can lower blood pressure. Here's how it works. First you say to yourself, "Now it's time to relax. You are going to go to a really restful place for a little while." No, I'm just kidding, you don't really *have* to talk to yourself in order to do this.

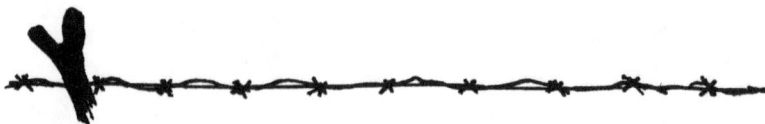

Sit in a comfortable chair with your feet flat on the floor. If you think that you might go to sleep, set an alarm so that you can be unconcerned about the time. Give yourself 10-15 minutes. Close your eyes and imagine yourself in a beautiful, very pleasant place, with no people. Choose a place you actually have been, or invent one that you would like to visit. Some people choose the mountains, beside a quiet stream. Others enjoy the beach. Now, picture that place, in detail. Besides the pictures you see in your mind, imagine the sounds you hear. Are there birds singing? Can you hear the surf rolling in? Is the wind blowing in the trees? Do you smell the perfume of wildflowers? Is the temperature in your imaginary spot pleasant to you? Explore the place as if you were relaxing there, moving slowly. There's no rush because you can go there again and again. Having some difficulty keeping the image in view? Don't be concerned. If you relax, it will come back. Breathe slowly and empty your mind of everything but the restful place you have chosen.

Just tell yourself to do it. If you think that learning relaxation methods sounds useful, but that you don't have time to take 10 or 15 minutes a day to use either method, then that is probably a sign that you really need relaxation to put yourself in condition to manage stress. You are the one who really *should* talk to yourself. Repeat after me, "I am going to practice a relaxation exercise every day."

—Teddy

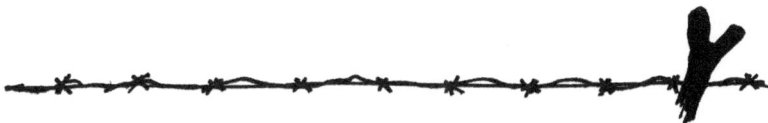

Capsule 35

Front Porch Chats

*L*ike many other families who lived on farms, my mother's family spent a great deal of time on the front porch. Swings and chairs provided opportunity for resting or socializing. My mom can still recall summer sleepovers on her front porch. They would drag the mattresses off the beds and have plenty of room on the porch to make their cots. The dogs would keep watch for any varmints or snakes so that a good night's rest was insured.

With air-conditioned homes today, a front porch isn't the coolest spot in a country home any more. Still, it's a convenient place for rural families to go and talk, and just like generations before them, the topic of conversation is often the weather.

How many of you who grew up on a farm or ranch can remember watching a parent or grandparent go stand on the porch to see if a cloud was coming up? An anxious father might pace the porch, or he might sit quietly offering a prayer. I suspect many a bargain has been made from front porch swings. Prayers go up that a shower will fall. But in another breath, there are prayers asking for no hail or high winds.

Since agriculture is such a large part of life in these areas, watching weather becomes second nature, no pun intended. Rainfall totals in the southwestern part of the United States vary as much as the weather. In East Texas some places may average over 50 inches a year. By contrast, some cotton fields on dry Texas plains see less than ten.

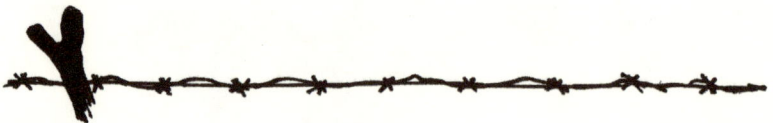

Tornadoes and hailstorms are another force of nature that frequents the South and Southwest just as snowstorms visit the North and Northeast. Perhaps other than earthquakes, nothing is better than tornadoes and other severe thunderstorms to impress upon us that weather predictions, though valuable, never allow us to control nature.

Often where there is a tornado there is hail, and to the farmer this is one of nature's cruelest tricks. It is moisture that is so needed, but hail usually takes more than it gives. If crops have just begun to produce, a hailstorm can wipe them out before they even start growing. Farmers are forced to replant.

Sometimes the hail comes late in the season, which is perhaps the most devastating. The work has been done, the stalks are high, and often the bloom indicates a bumper crop is on the way. A storm with just pea size hail, if intense and lasting longer than a few minutes can rip the stalks clean. In some places, hailstorms destroy a section of cropland and leave acreage two miles down the road untouched.

Because of their livestock, ranchers also are wary of storms that produce hail. Hailstones the size of baseballs, sometimes grapefruit, have been known to kill cattle that are basically unprotected in the pasture land. Ranchers might have time to get shelter for cattle, but farmers are totally at the mercy of the elements.

So why bother with weather forecasts and predictions? What good is it going to do? My theory is that between the 6 o'clock and 10 o'clock television weather reports, country folks know they have plenty of time to sit in their swings, drink some iced tea, and bargain with the heavens. It's called spiritual subsidizing and is a lot cheaper than cloud seeding.

If the clouds pass and it doesn't rain, there is still a silver lining to those storm clouds. Pull out the mattresses and sleep on the front porch, just for old time's sake.

—Sue Jane

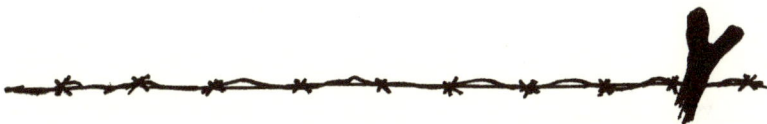

Capsule 36

Green Pastures and Still Waters

I get dogged tired sometimes. Too busy. Too scattered. Too few hours in the day to get done the things I need to do, much less the things I want to do.

I don't think this is a result of "the times we live in." I bet my grandmother, a widow at the age of 41 and rearing five children on a farm in the 1930s, had days like this, too.

My papers may not get graded, but she had to milk the cows and gather the eggs. I miss a deadline to turn in grade reports, but she had to pay taxes on time to keep the farm. I will go home after a ballgame and do some midnight laundry; she would come in from the fields after dark and do the same, but without a washer and a dryer. I won't even begin to think about cooking three hot meals a day. She did every day.

Grandmother McCleskey worked hard as farm manager and mother. She did so because she wanted her five children to have choices. My uncles made the choice to go serve in World War II. They came home after the war and attended college on the G.I. Bill. My mother and her sisters were able to attend college, too, because Grandmother went to bed dogged tired every night.

Sometimes, I have chosen way too much, and I'm not so sure my grandmother would have wanted me to run myself ragged. She was

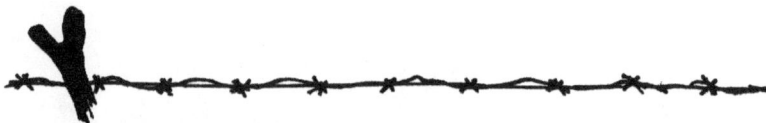

wise enough to know that rest was vital to not just the body but the spirit.

Grandmother took time in the afternoon and on Sundays to do something I often neglect to do: lie down, read the paper, and take a nap. Those were her green pastures and still waters in a life filled with hard labor, heartache, and loneliness.

Restoring our souls isn't always about gathering at a building to attend worship. It becomes a gift from above when we learn to take care of ourselves, and that's a choice we can all make.

—Sue Jane

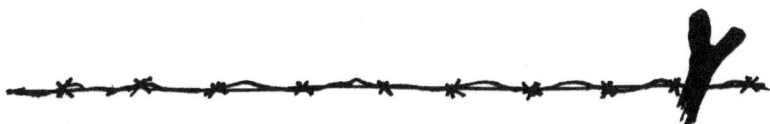

Capsule 37

Listen to This

No traffic passes today and seldom much on any day. Perfect driving. Pete Jones, the fast white dog, and I clip along in our red pickup. From the farm to the clinic in New Mexico where I'll see patients, we'll drive about 200 miles. The distance slides by and the scene changes. Leaving the high plains, we climb toward the mountains that appear on the horizon like a new set for the next act in a stage production.

Suddenly, I realize something has changed. The music has stopped. We're trapped in the space between radio signals. The Public Radio station in Portales is lost and there's nothing to replace it except a station with too much talk and too many commercials. No worries. The selection of recorded music rides with us. Pete can't operate the zipper on the tape case, yet, so I select traveling music. All is right again as soon as Willie Nelson begins singing "Phases and Stages."

That little episode set me thinking about music and its health benefits. I wondered, besides the fact that I enjoy music, is there any scientific basis for suggesting its use in health care? I vowed I'd look for an answer to that question.

Here's what I found. The answer is yes. In fact, the occupational field of music therapy focuses entirely on the use of music to promote healing. Research by music therapists, nurses, and others has explored the positive health effects of music. For example, use of music in hospice

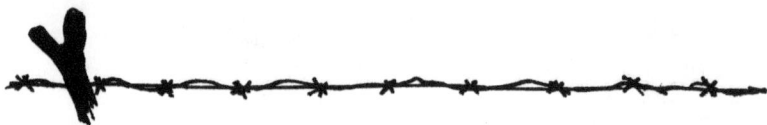

care benefited patients and their families. Cancer patients dealt better with pain and rated their quality of life as being better. Pre and post-surgical patients had reduced anxiety when they listened to music. Anxious and high stress patients showed lowered anxiety and reduced stress when music was part of therapy. Elderly persons showed improvement in balance and walking when their exercise program included music. Underweight newborns gained weight faster and Alzheimer's patients' behavioral problems improved with music.

It's not necessary to be ill for music to have value. Do you recall being a teenager? What music energized your adolescent moods? Would it surprise you that those same songs could perk you up on a down day even now? Hearing Elvis Presley sing anything he sang when he was handsome and I was 14 surely makes me smile. Or what about the energizing effect of a rousing march or the special feeling that church music prompts? Physiologists are not yet certain *exactly* what mechanisms create the changes in heart rate and blood pressure or muscle relaxation or the changes in neuro-chemicals and related moods that music apparently creates. But even without knowing exactly, we do know we can use music to our benefit. Let's not wait until someone is ill or having surgery to try it. Instead, focusing on health promotion, use music to encourage exercise, to promote stress reduction and relaxation, to block worrisome thoughts, and to encourage sleep. Here are some useful principles:

❂ Music you react to positively will be the most effective for you. Individualize. Use Willie Nelson or the Glenn Miller Orchestra if you want, but don't expect your 16 year-old relative to choose the same.
❂ Instrumental music is best for relaxation. Save the lyrics for exercise or to block worrisome thought.

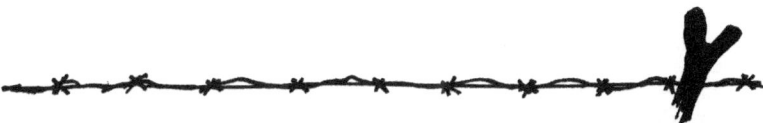

- Make your music easily accessible. If your old tractor doesn't have a tape deck, take along a portable and earphones. Carry a tune selection in the pickup. If you have special favorites, make your own tape or CDs for relaxation, for exercise, etc.
- Tempo and rhythm of the music should suit the purpose—upbeat and more rapid for exercise; slower, softer and flowing for relaxation.

As for the specific health promotion uses, music to encourage exercise can be selected to fit the exercise. A dance medley can accompany aerobics routines. Walking is more enjoyable with a march coming through your headphones. Relaxation, stress reduction and sleep encouragement are best aided by music that is slower, has little or no percussion, and calls to mind pleasant memories or calm moments. Worrisome thoughts can be blocked by various types of music, depending on your preferences. Music with lyrics I sing along to (Pete doesn't mind) works for me.

Even if there were no specific health-promoting benefits of music, our lives would still be enhanced by its presence. Whatever your preference of musical types, I encourage you to add more. Turn off talk radio, mute the TV, listen to music. It's good for your health.

—Teddy

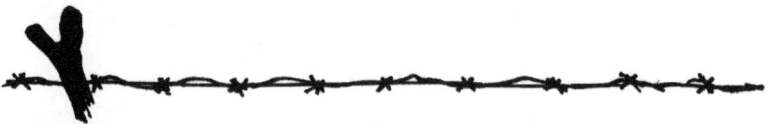

Capsule 38

Be Aware

I love the symphony, but I could not tell you the difference between "adagio" and "allegro." There is no real classical training in my background other than nine years of piano lessons. The ivories did not tickle me at the time.

I also love art. Museums, paintings, bohemian-type people fascinate me, but my knowledge of art does not go much beyond the good sense I have to spend a little more money on Crayola colors as opposed to the cheap brand.

As for fashion, I have none, but what I wouldn't give to have style like Diane Keaton. When it comes to dancing, my lack of rhythm gives me the blues, but I love to watch Gene Kelly movies.

And finally, there's singing. Ever since the kindergarten trauma of my stage-fright solo, I've appreciated those who can sing their songs as if no one were listening.

There's a word for people like me who appreciate (amateurishly) those aesthetically pleasing things in life—dilettantes. That just means I don't know squat about much, but it doesn't prevent me from being a big fan. And I can thank some great teachers in a small town for opening my eyes to a world of art and music and literature that can exist anywhere if one is willing to look.

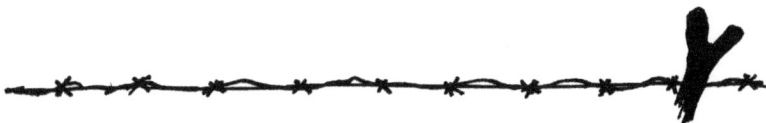

Miss Munson came to my hometown in 1970 to teach English at Travis Jr. High. It was my last year in junior high (9th grade) and her first year to teach at the young age of 21. She'd graduated early from college.

We girls in particular paid close attention to what she wore. From her, I learned that dressing well was a professional choice—and daily she came looking fresh and ready. The guys were more interested in her red Camaro, a vehicle that stood out on a small town campus among pick-up trucks, hand-me-down Buicks, and station wagons.

Young in years but blessed with travel experiences, a love of literature, and a passion for teaching, this young woman brought to our small world her knowledge and appreciation for music, art, and writing. It didn't hurt that she had a wonderful sense of humor that allowed for us to be sarcastic without getting in trouble. In the 1970s, many authority figures viewed a sharp wit as disrespectful; Miss Munson saw it as a higher level of thinking.

Her classes listened to and wrote poetry. She shared some of her own with us. It was the age of that Rod McKuen style, so we were not restrained with rhythm and rhyme scheme. We wrote our own, and she typed those poems and we put them in handmade books, our own publications in chapbooks bound in construction paper.

I never had a teacher play music in class before, but a record player with LPs was a fixture in hers. All kinds of music, too. Classical or Motown, we listened to a variety. Sometimes she would give us copies of lyrics and challenge us to find the literary devices we had studied.

A special bond grew that year between teacher and students; she and I stayed in touch through the years as I went on to become an English teacher, too.

I remember a letter she wrote me one time before I graduated. In it, she gave me some simple advice. So simple, it came in two words: be aware. Be aware of all the beauty that is around you, wherever you are.

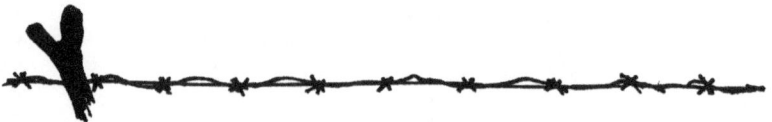

Rural communities where I now teach may have their fair share of rednecks, but I'm going to make sure mine are enlightened ones.

Teaching English and Spanish in a small, rural school often prevents opportunities for field trips to museums, but in my classroom there is an abundance of music and art. It's rather like I have taken up the gauntlet and vowed to bring the world to our little school.

On given days, we may listen to anything from Glenn Miller to Patsy Cline to Yo Yo Ma.

My students will also be exposed to both sides of the political fence so that they will think, not mimic. Small towns may not have major newspapers on handy racks, but with access to the Internet, I make good editorials available to my students by reading them aloud in class.

Sometimes, I have taken our little school out into the world. When money and time have allowed, my senior Spanish III students and I have traveled to Fort Worth (some five hours away) to go to see and hear symphonic performances at the beautiful Bass Hall. The Kimbell Art Museum provides a free glimpse at an original Picasso, Goya, and Miró.

Years ago I ran into an old high school classmate who asked me what I was doing. When I told her I was a schoolteacher at a small school, she seemed a little stunned and made the comment that she thought I had more ambition than that.

She was right about one thing—teaching is not about personal ambition.

Good teachers are more concerned about what they give rather than what they receive. Many rural schools are fortunate to have at least one teacher whose ambition is for his or her students to be aware.

What students choose to do with the knowledge and experiences the teacher exposes them to, whether they accept it or reject it, is their call. Real education is not about brainwashing either.

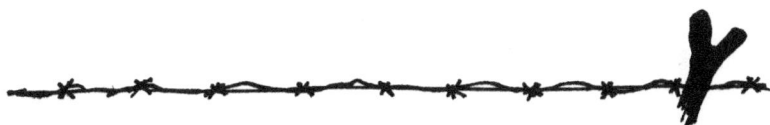

Miss Munson was one of the good teachers. The lesson she taught is one I still use everyday: that the size of the school or the community should never prevent exposure to an enlightened view of the world.

—Sue Jane

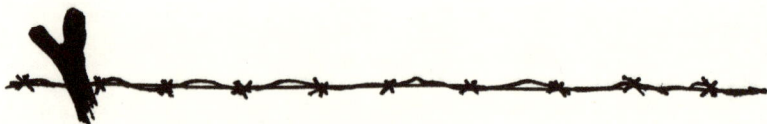

Capsule 39

Judging a Book by Its Cover

*B*ookstores fascinate me; this would probably not be unusual except for the fact that I am not an avid reader. I am a recreational reader, mainly nonfiction. So for me, a bookstore's not exactly like a candy store, where I indulge myself. But I know that literature is there for the taking, and it is perhaps that glorious offer in a bookstore that I find thrilling.

While visiting the Northwest last summer, a book I found seemed to invite itself home. I hate it when books do that. The book cover, the title, and image it conveyed about a woman's courage near the end of the 19th century convinced me to shell out a few dollars in spite of myself.

That night I began reading about Helga. The writing was not gripping, but the story certainly was. Helga became a heroine to me overnight.

Her trek across the United States in 1896 from Spokane, Washington to New York was a final attempt to save the family farm. If she could accomplish that feat in months, she would claim a $10,000 prize from an anonymous donor and save the farm.

Think about it. A woman walking—that was one of the requirements—more than 2700 miles, with her 18-year old daughter as her only companion except for the revolver she carried.

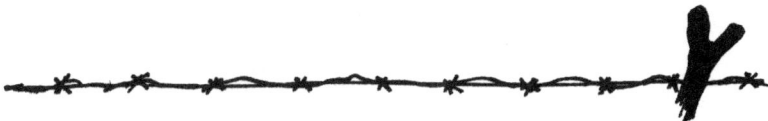

Desperate times were calling for desperate measures. Times like that exist for some today, and I wonder what stories are out there of women on farms and ranches in such straits. Helga responded to a desperate situation by accepting a challenge. Women today do the same thing, but unless those stories are told, they too will be lost. To survive in the future, we must know the past.

Ollie Holmes is one of my rural neighbors. She has farmed by her husband's side for most of their 40-year marriage. When Kent has suffered illness and couldn't work in the fields, Ollie's experience serves them well—she is not his hand but his partner. When Kent has to be away to teach voluntarily the county's EMT classes, Ollie does the farming. She also serves as Kent's secretary and types his EMT tests. Could Kent get by without Ollie? He would say no. Could she take care of the farm without him? That's a definite yes.

Does Helga do it? Does she win the money, save the farm, live happily ever after?

Read the book, *Bold Spirit: Helga Estby's Forgotten Walk Across Victorian America*. And every now and then feel free to judge a book by its cover. Learn the stories of the women in your rural areas who today carry some of Helga's bold spirit within.

—Sue Jane

 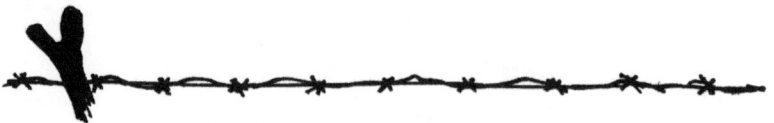

Capsule 40

Worship at South 40 and Mesquite

*There is nothing more important. With it, life is sublime;
without it, there is constant stress. It is the secret of true
greatness, the source of lasting happiness, the supply of
wisdom beyond our understanding, the strength to endure
in tough times, and the success in reaching what really
counts. It is our ultimate goal, life's greatest privilege.*

Lloyd Ogilvie, a chaplain in the U.S. Senate, shared these words in a 1998 speech entitled "Do You Know God?" Knowledge of God is the "it" to which he refers.

There was a time in my life when I thought knowing God meant the rituals, the motions, and of course, the attendance. Let me re-phrase that. I thought participating in those things was the *only* way to know God.

I am proud to say I have been healed. Healing is the correct word, too, because it has been through deep wounds that spirituality has emerged from what was largely religious doctrine. My maternal grandmother would know exactly what I mean.

Grandmother spent her life in the country. The church she attended in town was nine miles down a dusty, red clay road in Fisher County. She quit attending sometime in her mid-forties. Her reasons for "leaving the fellowship" as her mother and sister bemoaned require no explanation for me now. I have learned enough about my grandmother to know that her attendance drought did not affect what was in her heart.

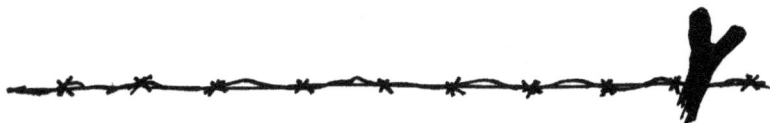

When a male tenant on her farm, also an elder in a church, pressured her to renege on an original agreement that would benefit him financially, Grandmother firmly and fairly refused. The tenant used his clerical position to turn other church members against her. They even paid her a visit to admonish her.

When she stopped going to church, family and friends reacted by making it a point to bring her back to the fold. Her mother and sister would drive by every Sunday and say "Bessie, you know you ought to be in church." My mother—not even ten years old—was invited to go, but she held her mother's hand, lending support and somehow sensing that she was going to be closer to God right there on the front porch.

The church elders never came again to pay a social visit or ask if this widow woman without a car needed any assistance. They made certain, though, that they came during revivals with the visiting preacher to make annual attempts to save her from eternal damnation.

"By your fruits, you shall know them."

Biblical principles of patience, kindness, and joy were the fruits my mother witnessed in her mother during those years when Sundays were spent at the farm.

Grandmother had patience with her five children. The four older ones assumed a great deal of responsibility on a farm that they were determined to hang on to after the death of their father. My mother, who was three months old at the time of her father's death, must have tested that patience as the youngest. But her recollection is that Grandmother allowed her the chance to do what the others could not do as often—enjoy childhood. She let my mother eat chocolate pie for breakfast, roam the canyon near their home, invite a best friend over for a sleepover on the porch, and play with dolls and games. Misbehavior, however, was exempt from the patience—Grandmother wasn't going to spoil her children.

She exhibited kindness often to her rural neighbors. No one really

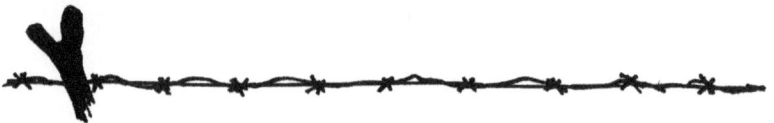

had money to spare in the 1930s, but a garden could provide nutrition in the difficult dust bowl days. She would pack homemade goods in a basket and take the wagon or walk with my mother in tow to a neighbor in need. It was a practical and natural kindness that the elders of the church should have imitated.

Above all else, there was joy. Mother remembers vividly her mother's laughter. Here she was a widow at 41 with a baby and four other children living miles from town, without a car, in the 1930s. Rather than wallow in the circumstance, Grandmother found joy being able to watch her children play on the few occasions they could. Grandmother delighted in playing Chinese checkers or dominoes or 42 with her children at night or on a rainy day when farm work wasn't possible.

Patience and kindness and joy were her living examples of faith. They tell me more about my grandmother than how often she went to church. She did not memorize verses to quote them; she knew them by heart so she could put them into practice.

In the early 1950s, after her children were all grown and gone, Grandmother started going to church in town again. The elders no doubt welcomed her and her money back with open arms. Her benevolence was instrumental in helping construct the church building that still stands in the small community today.

Some fifty years later, I find myself the beneficiary of her wisdom. For almost fifty years, my church home has been the same. My "family" there has witnessed my birth, my marriage, the birth of my children, my divorce, and my soon-to-be-empty nest. Through all those stages, their love and support has remained steadfast.

Sometimes, though not often, I choose to stay home instead of attending church services. I want to rest, to be alone, to study, or to write.

And my family knows I know God, the same God my grandmother knew so well.

As vital as human contact (fellowship) is to a person's well being,

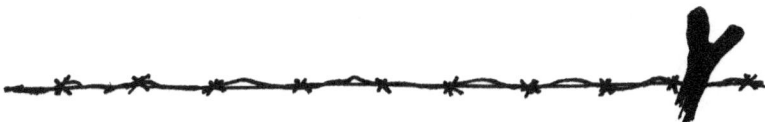

we can be detoured spiritually if the motive for that fellowship is short of anything other than knowing God better.

We may choose pews or we may opt for a Sunday drive. It really does not matter as much where *we* are but where *He* is.

From an old hymn that Grandmother probably sang at some point in her life, "Father and Friend, Thy Light" come these words which soothe: *Thy children shall not faint nor fear, sustained by this delightful tho't; since Thou, their God, art everywhere, They cannot be where Thou art not.*

—Sue Jane

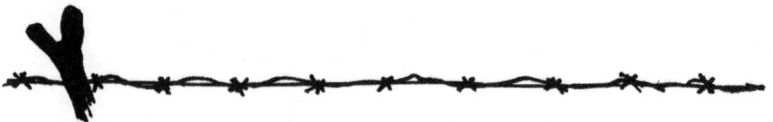

Capsule 41

I Never Had To Wear A Union Suit

*R*eading upside-down is a learned skill. Sitting across the dining room table from Mr. Jones as he leafed through a catalogue, practicing my "USD" reading skill, I deciphered a caption in the underwear section. The words: "Union Suit." Wow, that sent me back to my childhood! I was thankful, once again, that, unlike two of my cousins, I never had to wear a union suit. Their mothers outfitted them in the short-legged version of that "keep warm underwear" as soon as the first norther blew into Iowa Park each year. They required them to wear their union suits until spring, in the belief that they protected against all kinds of cold-related illnesses.

Maybe those ugly underwear items didn't ward off the flu, but they probably did help in one way. They kept their core temperature up. That's as important for farm and ranch folks today as it was for those unstylishly clad girls in the late 1940s. Hypothermia can occur rapidly and can have dangerous results.

Here's how it works. Technically, hypothermia occurs when the body's core temperature drops to 95 degrees F. or below. It is considered mild at 95; moderate at 93; and severe at 90. The core temperature is the internal temperature in the central portion of the body, where 98.6 is normal. The brain responds to reductions in core temperature first by shivering and reducing circulation to the peripheral portions of the body

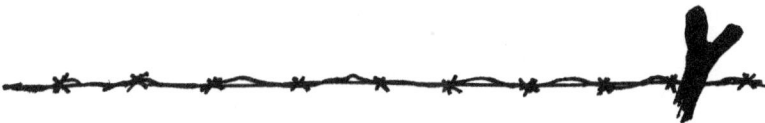

(feet, hands, face). That's why cold injury such as frostbite can occur with even moderate hypothermia. The circulation to those parts is reduced in an effort to keep the core temperature up, in order to keep vital processes of the heart, lungs, and brain operating.

"That's what the pickup's for," you're thinking. Good idea. But, I've seen people out breaking ice on stock tanks or trailing cattle that have wandered in a storm. And they were out of the pickup, in cold wind, for long periods of time. Or, haven't we all been stuck in icy mud on a turnrow or county road and had to dig out or walk in? It's not necessary to be a member of the Donner Party to risk hypothermia. It's a risk just going about your work when the conditions are right.

Factors can combine to create the conditions for hypothermia. It doesn't take a blizzard. Core temp can fall because of a combination of: temperature (the lower the greater the risk); wind; moisture (a wet body cools five times faster than a dry one and wet can be from snow, ice, rain, or sweat); clothing or lack of it; length of exposure to lowered temperature; general condition prior to exposure (poor circulation reduces the ability to respond to changes in temperature); and energy expenditures during exposure (a person who is exhausted is less able to generate internal heat).

As the body temperature declines, mental processes slow, decision-making is undermined and coordination is impaired. That's the perfect combination to produce accidents.

Prevention is more desirable than treating hypothermia or the result of an accident. Take these actions:

- Wear *layers* of clothing; remove and replace layers as needed to maintain a comfortable temperature at the chest.
- Wear gloves and warm socks; have spares along in case they get wet.
- Layer garments on the feet and hands for insulation also.

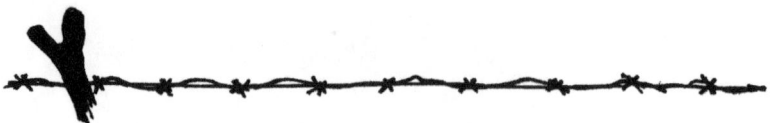

- ✪ Guard against getting wet. Keep a water repellent layer such as poncho and rain pants handy if there's moisture falling or you are working in mud or fallen snow; boots should be waterproofed or covered with galoshes.
- ✪ Rest periodically. The body's response to temperature reduction is to increase the metabolic rate. That tires a person. And the exertion of work increases the need for rest.
- ✪ Eat small amounts frequently. This provides "fuel" to help the body increase heat production.
- ✪ Drink warm liquids.
- ✪ Keep an eye on your companions. They may be unaware of their own condition as hypothermia affects judgment.

Those living in the Midwest, the northern half of Texas, or at high altitudes are more likely to risk hypothermia than those living south of Interstate 10. But, these same hazards are present in recreational situations popular in winter. When you "southerners" head for the ski slopes or for high country hunting, you should also remember your "union suits" and other methods for preventing hypothermia.

—Teddy

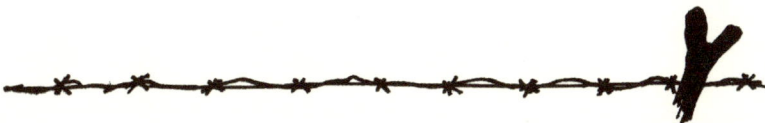

Capsule 42

I'll Take A Smiling Dog
Instead Of A Tranquilizer Any Day

*P*icture this. The Joneses (that's us) are driving the pickup on the north turnrow, doing 25 miles per hour. A white dog, with markings that look like she's wearing a black mask across her eyes, is running alongside, also at 25 miles per hour. The dog is smiling. I'm serious. This dog smiles. I believe it's because she knows that running is good for her health.

I'm smiling too, because I enjoy seeing her run so effortlessly. That's good for my health—the smiling, I mean. In fact, there is quite a bit of research that indicates that having a pet or even just interacting with a pet (without being fully responsible for the animal) has health benefits.

Here are a few examples of that research. One study showed that pets encourage social interaction between humans. This interaction is beneficial because it discourages social isolation. In that research, people passing by started conversations significantly more often with people who had a dog with them than when the same person had no dog. Apparently, something about the presence of the dog encouraged the contact between the humans.

Now, if the dog had been Pete (the fast white dog of unknown ancestry who runs beside our pickup) I *know* people would stop to talk—because *she* winks!

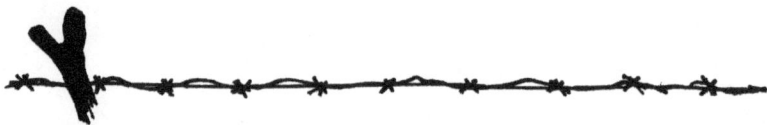

Several studies have confirmed that children who have responsibility for and attachment to a pet have psychological benefits from the interaction. Other research on adults has demonstrated a stress reduction benefit from holding and touching a cat or dog. Blood pressure and heart rate reductions, moving toward a relaxed state, were the measures that suggested stress reduction was occurring. Not all of the research has focused on dogs or cats as the pet. Birds, fish, and other creatures are "petworthy'" as well. Some of the benefits to humans who have pets seem to be related to taking responsibility for the creature and interacting with it regularly rather than just observing it. Responsibility for a pet requires daily attention. Some have suggested that there are health benefits prompted by having the pet as an external focus of attention, an important part of reducing anxiety.

Another human benefit from pet ownership is increased exercise. The exercise may be relatively little and somewhat repetitious, such as getting up from the chair to open the door for the cat to go out, come in, go out, come in, etc. Or, it may be more vigorous, such as the power walking required to keep up with Pete. Either is more beneficial than sitting still.

Of course, there are some cautions about choosing pets. These apply *if* a person has the opportunity to make the choice of pet. Until Pete, we had considered such things as size, activity needs and temperament when we adopted from the local animal shelter. But, Pete adopted *us* by jumping to the roof of our vehicle and refusing to budge when we started to leave the farm one day. We thought she was a stray. Apparently she was actually on a mission to adopt a family somewhere in Parmer County, Texas. So, we had no choice, it seemed.

Anyway, size of the pet should be a match for the person. A large dog is not a good choice for a small or frail human. Activity needs of the animal are important too. A fast dog like Pete needs someone who can move around pretty well. A less active pet such as a bird might

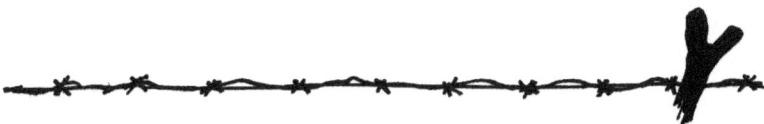

be a better choice for someone with mobility problems. Temperament of the pet owner should be considered also when selecting a pet. A person with limited patience may not do well with a young, less obedient animal or with a stubborn one like our previous dog, Lola the Bassett Hound.

Speaking of Lola, who died in an accident, reminds me of another health benefit that a pet can provide do for humans who are sad. When Lola died, Pete provided comfort to us. And speaking of Pete, she just stopped by to wink, smile, and tell me it's time to eat. Excuse me, I have to run get her meal!

—Teddy

 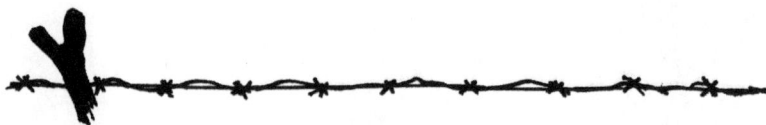

Capsule 43

Major, Collie and Queenie

*H*aving dogs around the house is nothing unusual for people who live in the country. Farm and ranch families know all too well that a dog serves many purposes. In fact, dogs could teach humans a few things about multi-tasking.

Major was my maternal grandfather's close companion on the farm in Fisher County in the late 1920s up until his death in 1931. When grandfather got the mules ready to plow, Major was at his side as if his job were to double-check the harness reins and serve as co-pilot.

After Grandfather died in an accident on the farm, Major went through the typical depression, not eating for a week. The first morning that my grandmother went to harness the mules and do the work her husband had done for years, Major knew it was time to transfer his loyalties.

That transfer of loyalty included not only Grandmother but also my mother, who was but three months old. Major's role expanded from partner to caretaker. He was to become a babysitter for my mother who was placed on a quilt in the shade near the orchard while Grandmother and her older children did the work on the farm.

In mother's infancy, Major kept bugs off the quilt and shooed the flies off the baby he was guarding. He alerted my grandmother if my mother cried. During mother's toddler years, Major adapted to her need

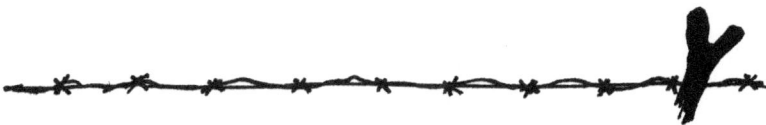

for some entertainment and on command to "Dig, Major, dig!" would do just that. He would dig a hole near the quilt, and Mother would playfully fill it up. Mother would have red clay on her hands while Major probably had some on his head where Mother would pat him in gratitude for a game well played.

He was also a protector. If someone other than Grandmother approached the quilt, Major's ears bent back and the inevitable growl left no doubt as to his intentions. Only Grandmother would be able to intervene and "call the dog off."

After Major died, my mother was given a collie that she named Collie. This breed was often used on the farm to herd up the cows for milking. Being the youngest in the family, Mother's job was to help Collie every day after school. Collie certainly bore the brunt of the labor as Mother often had to only say "time for cows." The cue was sufficient. It would be just a few minutes and soon Collie was running and nipping at the heels of the five or six milk cows that were being kept on the straight and narrow path to the fenced cow lot where Grandmother did the milking.

Collie, too, had another vital role. Uncle Preston and Uncle Clifton were Mother's two older brothers who did the typical big brother teasing from time to time. When Mother had enough, she would send her brothers scurrying for the fence with "Sic em', Collie." Little sister never hesitated to remind her brothers that she had an ally with big teeth.

Besides Major and Collie, my mother and grandmother had one more dog around the farm that quite possibly was the most talented of the three. Queenie was a snake killer. Snakes in this part of the country were a given, and Queenie seemed to have the instinct of a mongoose when it came to fighting rattlers.

Extremely protective of the women in the house, Queenie not only alerted them of the reptiles but also would "seek and destroy." She

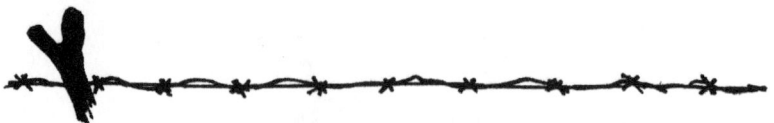

had a knack for knowing when to bite, watching carefully to see when the snake would retract to its coil. The mixed-breed dog then would grab the snake right below its head and sling it from side to side. If the dog's bite and whip-like tosses didn't finish off the snake, Queenie would repeat the process until the rattling ceased. She simply had no fear, maybe because she knew her role as protector.

As beloved as these animals were to my mother and grandmother, they were never allowed in the house. They never expected to be. Their domain was outside, and they monitored it day and night with faithfulness and loyalty.

After my mother left home to go to college, Grandmother had two more dogs. Skippy, a small mutt, and Mickey who was another collie, came to the farm. Years of needing a dog to baby-sit, to herd, to alert, or to protect were winding down. Now she just needed her dogs to keep her company. With age came mellowing, too. If anyone were to come by unexpectedly to visit Grandmother in those last years of her life, Skippy and Mickey came running *out* of the house to greet them.

The dynamics of all relationships change with time, even those between dogs and their owners. Grandmother lived long enough to experience the different bonds. After her death in 1955, the last two dogs ran away and never returned to the farmhouse. Somehow they knew their owner wasn't coming back, and more importantly, they understood that know one would love them quite the way she had.

—Sue Jane

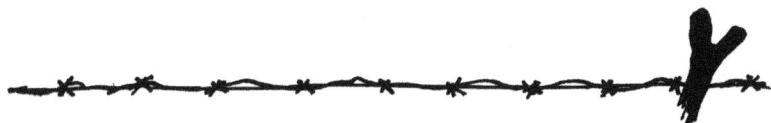

Capsule 44

Who Was That Masked Man?

"*A* fiery horse with the speed of light, a cloud of dust, and a hearty Hi-Yo Silver! The Lone Ranger rides again." Those lines came immediately to mind, along with that music, the William Tell Overture, as I a saw a neighbor wearing a mask while shredding his CRP acreage. The tractor didn't look much like Silver. Tonto was nowhere in sight. But, that farmer could qualify as "lone" because he is one of the few I have seen protecting his respiratory passages with a mask.

He isn't alone, though, in having a reason to breathe filtered air. Those most obviously in need of cleaner air are people with asthma. But, don't rule yourself out if you have never had asthma. Those who have hay fever, sinus infections, post nasal drainage and "summer colds" can also benefit from using masks. If you fit any of those categories or have family members who do, read on.

The entire respiratory tract including nose, sinuses, throat, trachea, bronchial tubes and lungs are covered by mucous membranes. (You are aware of that when the mucous cells begin to secrete gobs of runny stuff. "Where is all this coming from?" you exclaim in a voice that sounds canned.) Well, it is all coming from that mucous lining and it is being produced as a response to irritants or allergens that are inhaled. This is a protective response intended to keep the respiratory tract from being injured by the noxious item. We make mucous, we cough, we blow our

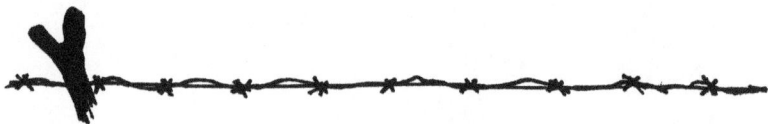

noses, it wears us out, but it starts out as protection for the sensitive respiratory tissues.

If you are allergic, any pollen you react to causes the response (and nose to run, etc., ad nauseum). Some people are allergic to grasses, some to weeds and flowers, some to trees, some to molds and some to all of the above plus many more things. It is difficult for a farm or ranch woman to avoid the plants that produce the offending pollens. And mold hides in the soil and loves to live in hay or in any dark, damp spot.

Even if you are not allergic, you encounter irritants that can prompt the same mucous result. Dust, cotton trash and gin residue, and grain chaff are examples of irritants that are almost impossible to avoid at certain times of the year. You plow, you harvest, you feed the animals.

An extra handkerchief would be all that is necessary if the excess watery secretion was the only reaction to breathing irritants or allergens. But there's another result in the respiratory tract when we inhale this gunk. The respiratory passages swell, holding more fluid in the tissues. This happens whether the cause is allergy or irritation. Then the tissues in the sinuses, those tiny air cavities associated with the nose, swell. The sinus becomes blocked, trapping the tide of mucous and any bacteria or viruses that might have strayed in there (with every breath- we're surrounded). Give them 24 hours and those critters start to multiply! The irritation or allergy has now been joined by a sinus infection! You recognize the infection by the colorful green and yellow of the secretions and the accompanying headache. You may have fever also.

To make matters worse, reaction of the lower respiratory tract to the allergen or irritant can cause that same type of mucous production and potential infection. If you are asthmatic, there is also an inflammatory reaction that starts the spasm in the bronchial tubes that you are unpleasantly familiar with. Put the upper and the lower respiratory problems together and you can be sick for days.

"Yes, but," you're probably thinking, "A mask is hot and looks

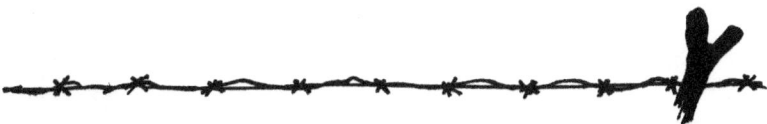

goofy besides." I can't argue with the part about it looking goofy. But you can take it off when you go to town. As for being hot, I would rather be a little warm than spend each night trying not to drown in post-nasal secretions. How about you? And, I have never enjoyed bronchitis a bit.

Another objection comes in the form of, "I'll just take sinus or allergy medicine to dry it up." Sometimes you will have to resort to that, but I'm talking about prevention, not locking the barn after the cow is gone. Besides that, most sinus medicine has pseudoephedrine in it, a drug that raises the blood pressure. Since commodity prices are enough to do that, it is better not to make matters worse.

If you are willing to try the mask, just pick up a box at the drug store. The molded ones made of micropore paper-type material are adequate for several hours' use each. They are inexpensive. They cost far less than a prescription for a sinus infection, bronchitis or a flare up of asthma.

Okay, so the Lone Ranger's mask was across his eyes—protecting his identity. Maybe he didn't need the nose and mouth mask. Maybe he never had allergies or sinus trouble. He probably never plowed a day in his life. And I doubt if he pitched hay for Silver, since his faithful scout Tonto took care of such chores. But, if he had done any of those jobs, I would have urged him to get a "real mask." I'm pretty sure he needed it, what with that cloud of dust that Silver created.

—Teddy

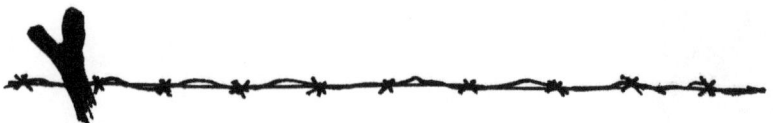

Capsule 45

If There's Anything I Dislike, It's A Smart Bug

*F*armers and ranchers are familiar with bugs. Some are beneficial. Some definitely are not. Some are microscopic; others visible to the naked eye. No, I am not about to launch into a treatise on how to combat Karnal Bunt or Hessian Fly. Nor do I plan to describe the best attack for Bovine Respiratory Disease. Rather, I want to let you in on some important information about "bugs" that affect humans. The news is—they are getting smarter!

According to the Centers for Disease Control and Prevention (CDC) the incidence of antibiotic resistant S. pneumoniae, common bacteria in the respiratory tract, has reached epidemic status. That means that those particular bacteria, which were in earlier times easily treated with ordinary antibiotics, have *changed*. They have evolved into "Supergerms" that no longer are susceptible to ordinary antibiotics. The sad part of the story is that we helped those bugs accomplish that genetic feat. How? We did it by using antibiotics to treat upper respiratory illnesses which were *not* caused by them and which were, instead, caused by viruses. You probably know that antibiotics do not kill viruses. And in most cases, our immune systems do a good job of handling the common ones. As a result, the S. pneumoniae which typically are carried by about 1/3 of young children and about 5% of adults, had the opportunity to

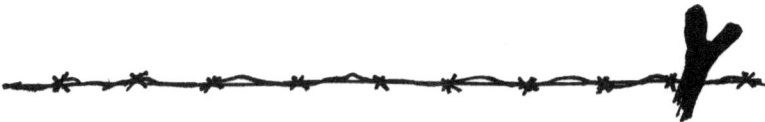

become resistant to those antibiotics. Those people who carry this germ are not made ill by it, but pass it to others in respiratory secretions.

First, those germs could ignore penicillin. Now, they are rapidly becoming stronger than many of the other antibiotic types as well. Next thing you know, germs wearing little Zs on their shirts will be taunting us saying, "This is what you get for using too many Z packs of Zithromax." The same series of events has occurred with some other bacteria as well, accounting for the development of life threatening illnesses caused by some staphylococci and streptococci.

As you read this, you probably do not have any respiratory symptoms. Maybe the usual cold, flu, and upper respiratory infection season has not yet arrived. And besides, what can you do about this anyway?

I am glad you asked.

The CDC, the American College of Physicians and the American Society of Internal Medicine have issued clinical guidelines urging physicians (and others who prescribe drugs) to be more discriminating in the decisions about treating upper respiratory illness with antibiotics. The materials they have distributed offer supporting research to convince health care providers that *in particular*, uncomplicated bronchitis, sinusitis, pharyngitis (sore throat), non-specific upper respiratory infections including the common cold, and flu do not benefit from antibiotics. In fact, the antibiotics create the possibility of side effects (such as diarrhea or yeast infections) and allergic reactions.

Certainly there are some people for whom an antibiotic would be important with a respiratory illness. For example, in those with chronic lung disease or other chronic diseases that reduce the immune system's strength, resident bacteria often create an infection when a virus taxes the immune system. Some sore throats are caused by Group A beta hemolytic streptococci which can be diagnosed by a throat swab test.

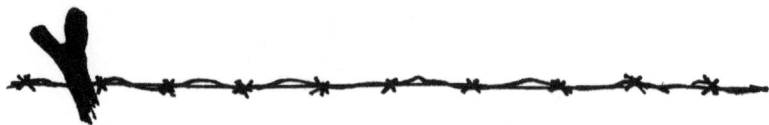

These infections need an antibiotic. But most sore throats are not strep, either in adults or children.

A person in agriculture knows that unnecessary inputs for crops and animal production are expensive and—well—unnecessary. You could think of unnecessary antibiotics in the same way—expensive and potentially damaging.

So, again you ask, "What can I do?"

Here's my answer. First, do not demand antibiotics for every respiratory illness. Nasal decongestants, fluids, REST, analgesics, and in some cases, a prescription bronchodilator inhalor will do wonders for symptoms while your immune system does the rest. Second, if your health care provider offers an antibiotic, ask if they think you really need it. "So, do you think this is viral or bacterial?" is a good opener for that conversation. Research has shown that many providers believe that patients will be dissatisfied if they do not get antibiotics. So, they have gotten in the habit of assuming that everyone wants one for an upper respiratory illness. Help them out. Show them you are a thinking person who wants antibiotics only if they are needed.

If we begin to reduce unnecessary antibiotic use, we can hope for decline in the incidence of serious illnesses created by resistant bacteria. We *can* be smarter than those bugs.

—Teddy

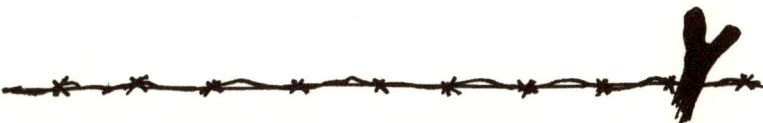

Capsule 46

Anything Worth Doing

*B*lack-eyed peas—two large grocery bags full, looks like a bushel—there they were waiting to be shelled. I started on them. It's mindless work, repetitive, leaving time for stray thoughts. And sure enough, here they came, those stray thoughts. It was the idea of repetition that came to me again and again. (Get it?) That led me to another health promotion concern, overuse injuries.

Those injuries of the musculoskeletal system are responsible for much pain, loss of work time, frequent medication use, and some surgeries. Among injuries in this category are carpal tunnel syndrome, tendonitis in various locations, bursitis, and muscle strains. Some of these injuries have colorful names like tennis elbow and housemaid's knee. They all have in common the fact that they often result from the stress of repetitive motion. In many cases, the repetitive motion is combined with poor body part alignment and bearing weight too great for the condition of the involved structures. The trauma of the repetitive motion and/or the strain of excess weight on the structure causes some combination of muscle fiber tears; inflammation of muscles, tendons, or ligaments or bursae; swelling; and pressure on nerves in the vicinity.

These injuries can be the result of movement required for work or for leisure activities such as sports or handcrafts. Common culprits in the work category you may encounter on the farm or ranch include

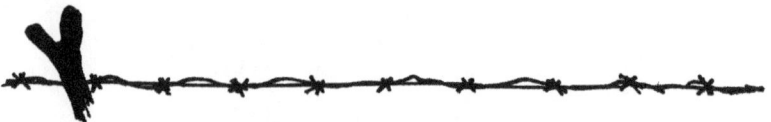

using a human-powered T-post driver; swinging a sledge hammer at any of the variety of items that require hammering; hoeing; roping calves; shelling black-eyed peas; peeling pounds of fresh peaches; lifting bags of feed ; lifting children; and making hand-sewn quilts. The list is endless. The point is that any movement that is *overdone* or improperly performed can cause an injury. You know it is an overuse injury when the soreness or stiffness does not go away in a day or two. If there is heat or swelling in the affected part or if numbness or tingling are associated with the body part, these are also symptoms of an injury requiring further care.

"But," you say, "I have a fence to help put up because there are cattle ready to graze the wheat pasture." "I have two quilts to finish before December." And I have those peas to shell. Well, the good news is that it is possible to prevent most repetitive motion injuries. Here are some principles to apply:

- ✪ Do stretching and light to moderate weight lifting regularly. Conditioning and warming up are crucial to all musculoskeletal activities. Daily stretching, for even a brief time, can provide both conditioning and warm-up for muscles and joint structures. Concentrate on hands, arms, shoulders, upper torso, hips and knees as well as stretches for lower back and legs. An entire routine can be completed in 15 minutes.

    There are many benefits to lifting light to moderate weights regularly (three times weekly). One of the major benefits is that when the muscle group are called into work, they are ready to bear the weight of a seven pound sledge hammer or a 50 pound grain sack. Ease into a program of stretching and lifting and stick with it no matter what your age or gender.

- ✪ Use tools and be certain they are well designed to reduce muscle strain. Tools of all sorts are intended as labor-saving devices. Look at the work you do and ask yourself if there are tools that

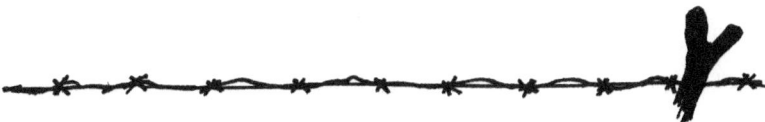

could ease the strain. For example, if you have seed sacks to unload, perhaps a dolly would be useful. If you shell peas very often, one of the nifty hand-crank shellers could be a boon. As for design, does your hammer fit your hand or does it need a larger handle? Considering tools and their design can reduce work and improve your efficiency while preventing injury.

- Check your posture as your work. Slouching in the tractor seat or at the computer can result in shoulder strain. Any awkward or poorly-aligned posture can create strain which, added to repetition of movement, can result in an injury. Sit and stand straight. Align the body for activity so that the strongest parts (leg and arms, not back) do the greatest work.

- Don't overdo! It is a temptation to do more, to meet a deadline we set, to finish just one more job, particularly when there is so much to do on the farm or ranch. Preventing overuse injury requires that we consider changing tasks to use different muscle groups rather than concentrating on a single task, resting occasionally, and recognizing the limitations of our bodies.

In case you are tempted to overdo, you might remember this: anything worth doing is worth not overdoing.

—Teddy

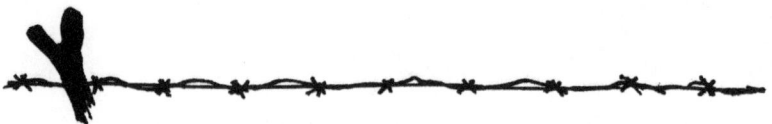

Capsule 47

Staying Too Close To The House?

"*I* thought you'd be over that respiratory infection by now, but I notice you've been staying close to home. Are you still sick?" A concerned friend is inquiring about his usual coffee drinking companion.

"Well, I haven't coughed in two or three days, but now I can't get far from the bathroom," came the reply.

His pal understood immediately and commiserated appropriately. He, too, had had experience with post-antibiotic diarrhea.

Necessary evil? Not necessarily. Here's what happens and some ideas about how to head off this aspect of the cure that sometimes is worse than the ill it treats.

Humans are the natural environment for lots of bacteria. Some of them are visitors of no special consequence that arrive on dirt, in water and in food. Some are potential pathogens that can cause illness if the immune system is not up to dealing with them. Still others are beneficial, serving useful functions in one or more regular body processes. These "beneficials" are similar in a way to the beneficial insects that live in certain crops. They help to keep the disease-causing bacteria population below illness-causing numbers. And they also play a part in some regular body processes. They're part of keeping the balance.

One such beneficial is Lactobacillus. This species normally inhabits the intestinal tract of humans, established there at the beginning

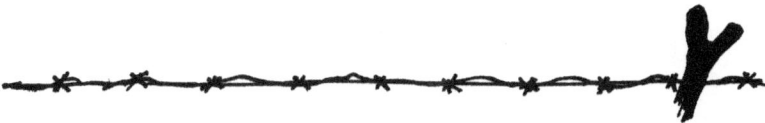

in the sterile intestine of the newborn through milk and subsequently through a regular diet. They arrive with the food, usually the dairy products. It earns its keep by fermenting lactic acid from carbohydrates-an important part of a dependable, orderly digestive process. Without lactobacilli—well, chaos ensues in the digestive process. You stay home a lot—close to the bathroom.

These naturally useful organisms can be destroyed when a person takes an antibiotic. Most antibiotics are somewhat indiscriminate in their bacteria fighting. Although they may be engineered to target certain bacteria more selectively, they are still more like a bomb than a rifle shot. They can do considerable collateral damage by wiping out the normal intestinal bacteria.

This is not peculiar to humans. Those who raise livestock and poultry or who "farm fish" may be familiar with the term "probiotics." These are bacteria that occur naturally in the animal under normal circumstances. Those bacteria are reduced or destroyed by antibiotics used to treat disease or by the conditions of production. These normal bacteria, when fed as a supplement, are called probiotics.

A probiotic to prevent or treat antibiotic-induced diarrhea in humans is easy to acquire. No prescription is needed. It's live-culture yogurt. You can use plain yogurt and add flavoring or buy the kind with fruit. But, be certain the package guarantees live culture. That means that the lactobacilli that make the milk into yogurt are still alive. Frozen yogurt doesn't guarantee the necessary live bacteria, so choose the regular yogurt. Eat a couple of ounces (more if you actually like it) three times a day as soon as you start taking the antibiotic. It works best if the antibiotics and the yogurt are separated by a couple of hours each time.

Since the yogurt is a pleasant tasting food, supplying lots of calcium and protein, there's no reason to wait for the diarrhea to start. Just take it as soon as you start the drugs and think of it as the more pleasant part of your treatment. If you really dislike yogurt, you can buy

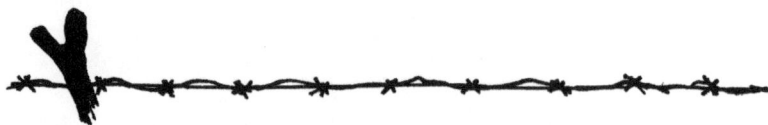

acidophilus capsules or tablets to supply the bacteria. These may be stored in the refrigerator rather than on the shelves at the pharmacy, so you might have to ask for them. However, the yogurt is far less expensive and has the added nutritional benefit. Either should be taken for as long as you are on antibiotics. The yogurt is safe for children as well as adults.

This preventive remedy sounds rather like common sense, but it is important to check to see if there is research to support its actual benefit. I found reported research that did demonstrate a reduction in antibiotic-induced diarrhea with the use of lactobacilli. However, there is advertising that markets the lactobacilli (acidophilus) tablets and capsules with claims that they should be taken daily (whether taking antibiotic or not) to stimulate the immune system. So far I have not found supporting research for these claims.

One caution is important in regard to antibiotic-induced diarrhea. In a small number of people, certain antibiotics have caused pseudomembranous colitis, an inflammatory process in the colon that requires other treatment. In these cases, simply replacing the bacteria is not sufficient. For this reason, if diarrhea (defined as numerous, not just loose stools) continues more than seven days while taking lactobacilli with the antibiotic, see your healthcare provider and be certain to mention that you have already used these beneficial bacteria.

—Teddy

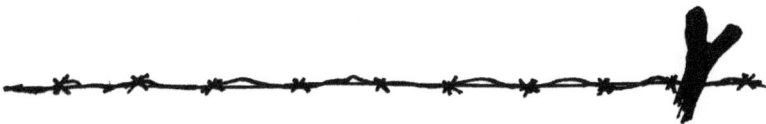

Capsule 48

Put Your Foot Down, But Gently

I won't say exactly why I was at the beauty shop, reclining with my neck on the rim of the shampoo bowl. Some things are private. But, I did learn that day that the local salon is another good place to hear some interesting things, especially if you have your eyes closed and keep your mouth shut.

"I woke up and started to get out of bed and the next thing I knew, well I nearly fell down. There was this pain that felt like a red hot poker in my heel," someone was saying.

"Was it a stone bruise?" asked a voice from a chair across the room. "I'll bet you have a heel spur," came from the front of the shop. I wanted to offer a bad joke, something like, "I bet that makes it hard to make a firm point, you know, to put your foot down." But, I thought better of it. My procedure was soon finished and I opened my eyes to see that the other patrons were gone. There I was with no one to give advice to. So you will get it instead.

That sudden heel pain that is worst immediately upon arising and continues as long as you are on your feet is characteristic of plantar fasciitis. The cause of the ailment is microscopic tears in the tissue that connects the heel to the base of the toes. It can be the result of a direct injury from stepping hard on something like a rock. That's why it has been sometimes identified as a stone bruise. But, more often, it is the

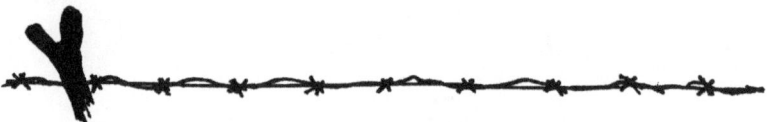

result of repeated strain on that tissue, the plantar fascia.

A strain of that type can happen easily in runners or other athletes. But it can also occur in people who stand or walk for extended periods, particularly if one is overweight or has flat feet. People whose calf muscles are very tight also more easily develop plantar fasciitis. And for some reason that's not clear, it occurs more often in females.

One line of thinking is that if this condition becomes chronic, the base of the heel bone responds to the inflammation by generating new bone cells as an attempt at protection. These are the "heel spurs" that you might have heard of. But, the heel spur development is not nearly as common as the inflammation.

Well, you've got work to do. There's no time, except maybe the dead of winter, when farm or ranch people can just sit around with their feet up. Are you going to have that pain every day from now on? Not necessarily. For a lot of people, the natural response of favoring the affected foot by limping, walking more on the front of the foot, will allow the inflammation to heal. But, doing nothing is probably not a particularly good idea since favoring one foot can cause strain and other problems with the knees or lower back. Everything is connected!

If you visit your health care provider, you will probably receive advice to, 1) take an anti-inflammatory medication for a couple of weeks, and 2) wear shoes with good arch support and a slightly higher heel to reduce the strain on the fascia. Gel heel inserts in the shoes can also accomplish the lift and can cushion the inflamed area. Some also suggest taping the arch for support or wearing a splint at night to flex the ankle and gently stretch the fascia without weight bearing. For cases that extend more than six months, some providers may use steroid injections directly into the heel or might recommend surgery. Others use external sound-shock wave treatment, the same as the method that breaks up kidney stones using sound waves transmitted through water.

Another important activity that is both treatment and prevention

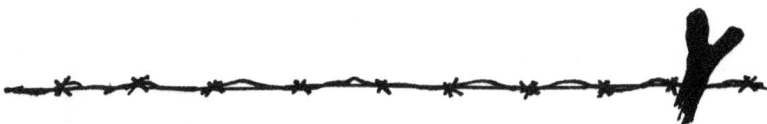

is stretching. Yes, that again. Before putting the foot on the floor the first time in the morning, flex the foot upward several times to loosen the muscles and the fascia. Then each day add the following stretch to your regular routine. Stand facing a wall, about three feet out. Keep the affected foot flat and the knee straight. Step forward on the other foot, bending the knee and leaning forward to touch the wall. Feel the stretch in the affected foot, Achilles tendon and calf muscle. Hold the position for 15 seconds. Repeat twenty times. For balance and prevention, do the same with the other foot.

The final part of dealing with this type of heel pain is to have patience—for two reasons. First, it often takes months for plantar fasciitis to resolve completely. And second, if you are impatient, you could be tempted to "put your foot down." Ouch.

—Teddy

 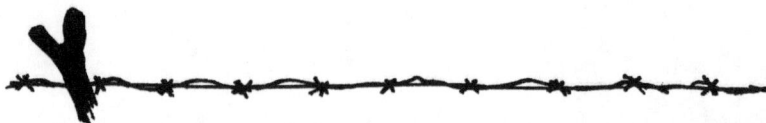

Capsule 49

It's A Pain In The...

*J*ust a little uneasiness in the middle of the chest, a bit of pressure. Then it increases; this is *pain* and increasing pressure. You check for other signs—no pain in the arms or neck, but this is a serious chest pain. You feel sort of clammy and your heart seems to skip a beat or to race. It doesn't go away. Next thing you know, you're in the Emergency Department. Tests are performed to rule out "all the usual suspects," including heart attack, gall bladder disease, and lung problems. Then someone in hospital garb hands you a glass and says, "Drink this please." The relief is quick. You've just had a "G.I. Cocktail." The combination of antacid, smooth muscle relaxant and topical anesthetic coats the upper gastrointestinal (G.I.) tract, relieving the symptoms handily. You may feel a little embarrassed, thinking, "What a pain in the..." But there's no need for embarrassment. It was real and will likely reoccur unless something is done to correct the problem.

The source of the pain was somewhere between the top of the esophagus and the bottom of the stomach. Gastroesophageal reflux, GERD, is a likely cause. Simply put, it means that the acid that the stomach produces to digest food is irritating the area at the bottom of the esophagus. That area is intended to be a one-way valve and is supposed to stay closed, except when you swallow. Some people may have only irritation, from too much acid. Others may have a "loose valve" that

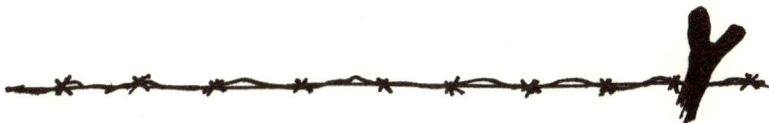

allows the acid to run uphill-up the esophagus. Still others may have a hiatal hernia, a protrusion of part of the stomach above the diaphragm, the muscle separating the chest from the abdomen. Any or a combination of these situations can cause severe pain. The irritation from the acid can also cause erosion and scarring of the esophagus. What's next? you wonder.

Of course, your medical history and other symptoms determine whether other tests are needed. But the likelihood is that one thing you'll receive is a prescription for a medication to reduce gastric acid. There are three classes of these drugs. Each class has a different action. Antacids such as Tums or Rolaids neutralize the acid *after* it's produced. Histamine-2 blockers cut down on acid production by blocking a part of the stomach chemistry that produces acid. Tagamet and Zantac are names you may recognize. The newer drugs, proton pump inhibitors, inhibit a different aspect of acid production. They include Prilosec, Nexium, Aciphex, and Protonix.

Newer is not always best, because different drugs will work for different people. But any of them work better for GERD if preventive steps are taken to reduce the acid production and to discourage any upward flow of stomach content.

Since prevention is my theme, I'll tell you some of the steps you can take. You might be surprised that these may relieve the need for medication. First, adjusting the diet can reduce acid production. Several foods and beverages are known to increase stomach acidity. They include alcohol, coffee and caffeine-containing drinks, onions, garlic, peppers, chocolate, nuts, peppermint, and fatty or fried foods. You might find that only some of these cause problems for you. Eliminate or reduce those that do. Second, stress also increases stomach acid as does nicotine use in all its forms. You can make changes in those, too.

Next, an empty stomach has nothing for the acid to work on compared to one with food in it. Does that mean you should eat more?

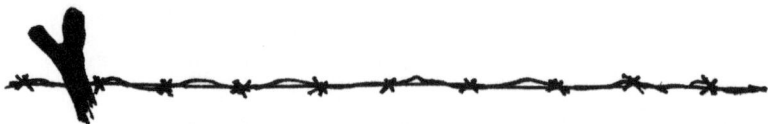

No, it means that dividing your food into five or six small meals a day can give the acid something to work on. Also, reducing the size of meals reduces the upward pressure on the esophagus that a full stomach causes. That full-stomach pressure is even worse if a person goes to bed full because lying flat makes it mechanically easier for the reflux to occur. Extra weight also promotes reflux because abdominal weight increases abdominal pressure. Lose weight. Reduce pressure. Reduce reflux.

Finally, elevating the head of the bed 6-8 inches by means of blocks placed under the bed frame will create a slight incline and discourage reflux.

—Teddy

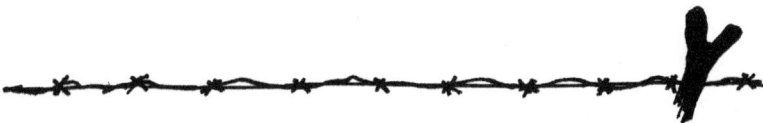

Capsule 50

Not In Polite Company

You'll hardly ever hear it mentioned at the Dairy Queen. No one's discussing this at the elevator or the gin. Seldom does the conversation at the beauty shop turn to this topic. We don't consider it a subject for polite company. And the biggest problem of all is it's too often not even mentioned within the family or to health care providers. Could be it's time to bring it up. Urinary incontinence. That's the *it* I'm talking about.

If the involuntary leakage of urine was discussed in polite company, you might be surprised how many people have to cope daily with the problem. Wonder why we keep it a secret and assume there's nothing much that can be done to help? Maybe folks believe that being unable to control urine flow is shameful. They manage in the only ways they know—by using "stay dry" garments, by ignoring odor, by staying home to avoid public accidents, or by suffering the isolation that staying out of polite company creates.

An estimated 15-35% of all non-institutionalized people older than 60 have some incontinence. But it happens to younger people too. Women are twice as likely as men to be affected. Fewer than 50% of those with leakage ever report it to their health care provider.

Besides the problems of isolation and distress created by urinary incontinence, other results are an increase in falls in the elderly and

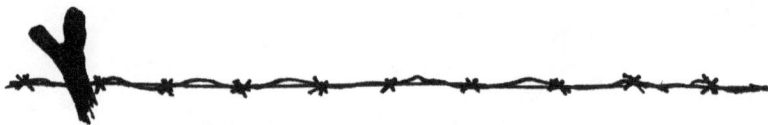

admissions to nursing homes. Why? The falls tend to happen when the incontinence is related to sudden uncontrollable urges to urinate. Hurrying to the bathroom, the person loses balance or slips. Falls decrease one's confidence in the ability to manage all daily activities. Worse, they can cause fractures or other injuries. You can easily see why admission to a nursing home can seem like the only solution.

Causes of incontinence include: 1) poor pelvic muscle tone and anatomical changes creating bladder pressure and poor outlet closure, 2) overactive bladder muscles, 3) neurological problems associated with illnesses that create reduced awareness of urge or which allow overfilling of the bladder, 4) medication side effects that create one of the previous three causes, or 5) a combination of two or more of these causes.

The most common cause in females is the first mentioned above. Poor pelvic muscle tone and structural changes are often associated with having been pregnant and having had a vaginal delivery. Menopause-related reduction in estrogen is also known to affect pelvic muscle tone. In men, prostate problems can create similar leakage. The term for this type of incontinence is *stress incontinence*. Some types of activity can increase bladder pressure. Coughing, sneezing, jumping, running and straining are examples. Structural changes caused by anything that increases abdominal and/ pelvic pressure (obesity, tumor, constipation, for example) can also create the physical stress that results in leakage when the muscles which close the bladder opening are weak.

The *overactive* bladder may cause frequent uncontrollable urges to urinate. The incontinence results because of the suddenness of the urge. Bladder infection is one cause of overactivity.

The bladder that is *underactive* overfills or never empties completely. Leakage results from the overflow.

Avoiding dealing with incontinence won't make it go away. Nor will simply thinking that it's part of aging prevent some of the negative results. There are several methods to treat and/or prevent incontinence.

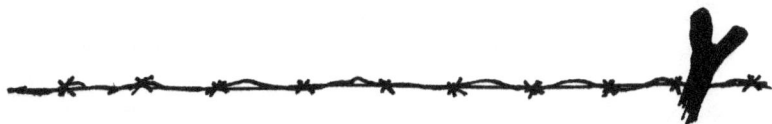

Depending on the type of problem, help may include changing, adding, or stopping a medication; doing daily exercises to strengthen pelvic muscles; training oneself to a schedule of urinating; eliminating caffeine from the diet; or treating an infection or constipation. In some cases surgical procedures can help.

I doubt that incontinence will ever be a common topic in polite company. But, it should be reported to your health care provider. The health care provider should investigate to pinpoint the cause. You can help by having facts. Those facts include when the problem began and an accurate description. Keeping a log for a couple of days will help. List the time and anything that seems associated (for example, coughing, waking from sleep, drinking three cups of coffee, pain, bleeding, etc.). Consider the mention as part of preventing the negative results, not as complaining about an embarrassing problem.

—Teddy

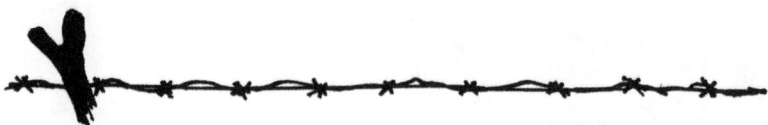

Capsule 51

Beneficials Or Boll Weevils?

*T*here I was, eavesdropping at the post office. "What is that little thing crawling out of my mailbox, Charlie? Is it a boll weevil come to town?"

"It's a ladybug, Marvin. Can't you see that?"

Good manners demanded that I move along, so I did not hear the rest of the conversation. But I imagined a joking discussion about Marvin's lack of visual acuity. It wouldn't be surprising since he appeared to be past 50 and was not wearing glasses.

All of us can expect our eyes to change as we pass 40. We just have to accept the fact that if we age, our eyes do, too. Presbyopia (the medical name for aging eyes) results from changes in the small muscles that constrict the pupil and in the lens. As the muscles respond more slowly to changes in light and the lens becomes less pliable, it takes longer for the eye to respond to changes in focus. We seem to need more light to get a sharp image. The letters dance off the page and our arms need extensions to hold what we want to read at the proper distance. Distance vision becomes less clear as well.

Another fairly common change in the eye that comes with age is cataract. That is where the lens (just behind the iris and pupil) becomes cloudy. The lens functions to concentrate light on the retina so that we perceive an image. The cloudiness of the lens causes the light to be less

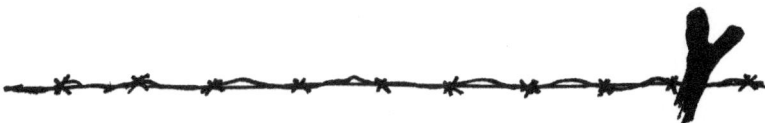

concentrated so the images become blurred and cloudy. That blurry vision, particularly in distant focus, is the first sign that a cataract is developing. Cataracts can be the result of harsh ultraviolet exposure over years and can be accelerated by smoking and by diabetes.

There are many problems caused by reduced vision from these two causes. For example, misreading can cause miscalculation in our checkbooks. The enjoyment of reading is reduced to the point that some people just quit. As vision fades, we can miss the beauty of our environment. With all of that, the quality of life is reduced. More serious are problems such as falls and driving accidents.

Maybe you've heard the tale about the old timer whose pickup collided with the preacher's car at the grocery store one day. The preacher was surveying the damage, after assuring that the senior citizen was not injured. He was puzzled when the older man said, "I called ahead."

"Do you mean you called ahead to let someone know you were going to visit?" the minister asked. "No," replied the senior driver, "I called to let everyone know to clear the road. I can't see past my nose."

Even though eyes change as we age, I don't much like the only alternative to growing older. So, the next best thing is to do what can be done to prevent what is preventable.

First, after the age of 40, even if we have never worn glasses before, we should all have an eye exam every year. If there are no problems other than presbyopia, the exam does not have to include dilation of the pupil each year. If you are diabetic, the annual eye exam should be with dilation.

When the first bifocals are prescribed, expect to feel some loss— youth is officially gone. Think of it this way—these bifocals come with the age that can signal that wisdom is arriving. Don't be surprised if the bifocal prescription changes every year or two until sometime between 60 and 70. The eye continues to change for about that long. Even after that, the exams need to continue to check for other problems.

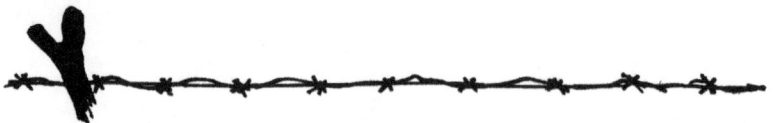

Wearing sunglasses is a good preventive step. The reduced exposure to the sun's ultraviolet rays can delay the potential for developing cataract. Research reported in 1994 suggested that a daily multivitamin supplement can reduce cataract risk. And other experts encourage a diet high in vitamins A, C, and E for the same reason. That's just one more reason to eat a diet that includes daily "doses" of fruit and yellow and green vegetables.

Back to my imagining again. I replay the conversation I heard. But, this time, Charlie looks different as he gives his reply. He is wearing bifocals and has some fashionable sunglasses clipped on them. "Marvin," he begins his reply," When you can't tell a boll weevil from a beneficial, it's time for you to get glasses. Let me give you the name of a good eye doctor. In fact, I'll drive you to your appointment so you won't have to call ahead!"

—Teddy

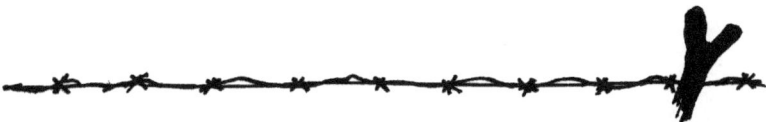

Capsule 52

On Balance

*H*ave you been there recently—in a heap on the floor or ground? Though it is said that walking is nothing more than controlled falling, the difference between upright and unintentionally horizontal is vast. It has to do, in part, with balance. It takes a complex combination of body parts working together to keep us on balance and standing. The inner ear, eyes, muscles, bones, several parts of the brain and the sensory and motor nerves tell us our position and maintain our posture and movement. It's an amazing concert of functions that lets us move about on two legs. Malfunction in any part can threaten the ability for balance and movement.

Falling seems easy enough for toddlers. They usually look surprised, bounce on their diaper and go on. After all, there's not far for them to go as they meet the ground. But as we grow, falls become, at the least, an embarrassment. If we do it often, we learn to think of ourselves as clumsy. And as we age a bit, we recognize that some danger is involved in taking a tumble. Most people, not including bull riders, do not voluntarily choose to fall. The possibility of adding injury to the insult of the embarrassment becomes an even greater concern when a person is less flexible in the joints and muscles or when bones are brittle.

"Ah," you think, "that leaves me out. I don't have osteoporosis

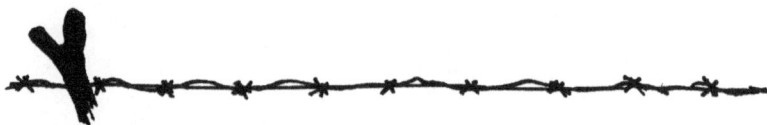

and I am young, strong and flexible." It's true that a younger, more flexible person is less likely to fall. But, even if this applies less to you than to your parents, I hope you will read on. Even the young and nimble can be prone (bad pun intended) to falls under certain conditions.

I won't dwell on all the possible results of falls. None of them is pleasant. They include bruises, sprains, strains, and fractures and the resulting need for some degree of immobility and inconvenience while healing. Another, more subtle, result is the erosion of confidence, the insult to one's sense of competence.

Conditions that predispose to falls are many. I have special titles for some of the more noteworthy. Each of those phrases describes a preventable cause of falls. Let me explain those causes and the prevention.

"These Shoes Are Made For Falling." The best shoes for preventing falls are those that provide a wide base. Flat heels are better than spikes and shoes with laces, buckles, or other closures are better than slip-ons. The worst footwear for contributing to falls are slides or backless *slippers*. (There's a reason for that name!)

"Who Moved That Rug? How Did That Table Get There?" Poor vision and poor light are more likely the culprits in this case than are furniture moving gremlins. Prevention? Regular vision exams, wearing the glasses if they are prescribed, cleaning eyeglasses regularly, and turning on adequate lights to see edges (of rugs and furniture) clearly are small, but important, preventive actions. About those rugs—there's a reason they're called throw rugs. They will—throw you.

"I Was Able To (fill in the blank) When I Was 20 (or 30 or 50)." Attempting activities that we do not have the strength, balance, or skill to perform accounts for many a tumble. Prevention in this case means staying in the best possible physical condition, with regular exercise for strength and flexibility. It also requires approaching any unaccustomed activity with a realistic notion about our abilities. A person who has not

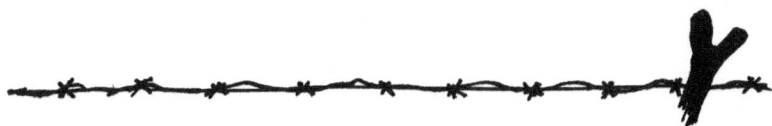

skied in 20 years should prepare with conditioning exercises. One who has not been on the roof for a while should approach the ladder reverently.

"This Medicine Works Great, But There Is One Side Effect." The side effect that causes a person's blood pressure to be lower when standing than when sitting or lying is most often implicated in falls. Don't do without your diuretic or blood pressure medicine. But do practice rising slowly from sitting or lying when you take any drugs that your pharmacist says can cause postural hypotension.

"The Next Thing I Knew." This implies a lack of awareness of one's surroundings, of hazards, or of one's actions. It doesn't mean anything particularly drastic, like being comatose. Rather, it reflects how we are when we are fatigued, preoccupied, or under stress. Those situations, as surely as throw rugs or medication, can put us "off balance." Prevention for this hazard is more complicated than for any other. It requires making a commitment to focus on one thing at a time, to recognize and take action to manage stress and to rest when we are tired.

Preventing falls is about staying balanced in every way.

—Teddy

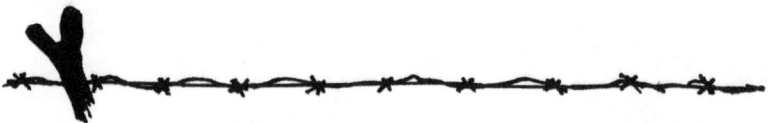

Capsule 53

I've Stopped Hoeing!

*H*oeing weeds is, for me, a satisfying activity. It's exercise for several muscle groups. It is performed outdoors. It releases frustrations and reduces stress. There's never a shortage of weeds to hoe. It's always there when I want to do it. It's good honest labor.

But, I've stopped hoeing because some time a while back, I overdid it. Must have made a muscle strain or a tendon inflamed or some other overuse injury. Assured by my health care provider that there's no other pathology in my upper back, left side, I had a choice. I could take medication (anti-inflammatory) or I could stop hoeing and let it heal. Actually, the health care provider didn't present the choice. She just said, "We could try one of the new anti-inflammatories (then mentioned the name of the latest drug spelled with an X to make it sound powerful). Shall I write you a prescription?" I said, "No, but thanks." She moved on to the next subject.

I like my primary care provider. I believe she's up-to-date and interested in doing a good job. But as I thought about that encounter, it occurred to me that the same type of conversation goes on every day in clinics everywhere. And that type of discussion accounts for a part of the increase in the use of prescription and non-prescription drugs.

In far too many of these clinic visits, the option to recommend what the health care literature calls "lifestyle modification" is either

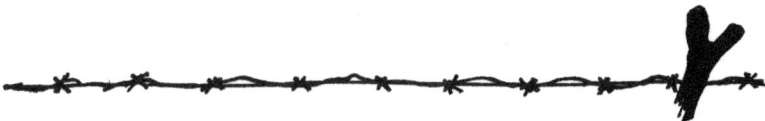

omitted or is given little emphasis. At the same time the use of medication is standard practice.

I have no research to support my opinion, but here's why I think this happens. First, many health care providers truly believe that medication is what the patient wants and that if no prescription is given, the patient will be dissatisfied with their care.

Second, perhaps patients *do* want medication. It's an easier and quicker fix (sometimes), if you have the money to buy the drug. Advertising by drug manufacturers encourages us to believe that almost any condition, even the simplest of ills, is best remedied by use of medication. Anyone who reads newspapers, magazines, listens to radio or watches TV could easily accept that idea.

Third, health care providers may have learned from their experience that people disregard advice about lifestyle modification. So they decide not to waste their breath explaining the non-medication possibilities.

Lifestyle modifications are changes and we all know that change is difficult. But, if the choice is between making a change in exercise or diet or in some aspect of our living arrangement versus taking medication, maybe it's worth considering.

Before I continue, and lest I be misunderstood, I am *not* against the use of medication. In some cases, and for some illnesses, it's absolutely necessary to take medication. However, there are many situations where taking charge and making a change in our behavior can eliminate the problem.

One example of such a situation is mild hypertension. When slightly elevated blood pressure is detected, current treatment standards say that if there are no other risk factors, there should be a trial of lifestyle modification. That's where the patient should receive information about what changes in weight, exercise, stress reduction, and diet they should

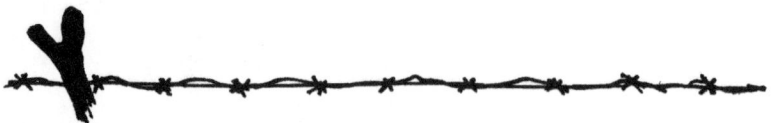

begin. Then they should be monitored. If the changes are not effective, medication is next.

Another example is hyperlipidemia. Elevated cholesterol, low HDL (High-Density Lipoprotein), high LDL (Low-Density Lipoprotein), and high Triglycerides can be changed with diet and exercise modifications *in some patients*. Treatment guidelines state that these changes should be recommended. Again, the advice must be specific and targeted to the individual patient.

Treatment for Gastro-esophageal Reflux (you may call it bad indigestion) can include an initial trial of changes in diet and meal schedules along with simple over-the-counter antacids. But the ads in the media tell you to "ask your doctor for the purple pill."

With the costs of medication increasing every year, the issue of cost alone makes it logical to take this personally. What can we do?

First, begin to think seriously about whether you expect medication to "do all the work". Would you be a dissatisfied patient if your "prescription" was specific direction about lifestyle modification rather than a medication?

Second, actively encourage your health care provider to give you the specifics about what you should modify. Practice asking questions like, "Are there things I should change that could keep me from needing a medication? I'd really like to give that a try." Or you might say, "Do you have a brochure or other material to tell me more about how to reduce whatever makes my triglycerides high?"

And, if you already know what you need to do—you can just stop hoeing.

—Teddy

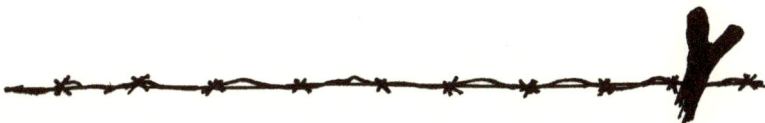

Capsule 54

It's Not The Age, It's the Mileage, Or Maybe Something Else

*S*omeone told me that the older we are, the more time it takes to do all the necessary maintenance just to keep ourselves in working order. There's some truth to that. I've also observed that there's a tendency to attribute a lot of pains, aches, and general ill-feeling to age or "mileage" that may not be related to either one. There's no rule that a person has to feel worse every day after age 35. And if we tend to preventive maintenance, the mileage won't necessarily create daily misery.

So, when those vague changes that too often are attributed to age or mileage occur, investigate before settling for those easy but distasteful answers. Here's just one example. Trouble concentrating? Fingernails brittle? Tired a lot? Gaining weight? All those symptoms could be attributed to aging or to just being run down. But they also could suggest a common condition that often goes undiagnosed, hypothyroidism.

There are two general types of malfunction of the thyroid, hyperthyroidism (over-production) and hypothyroidism (underproduction). It's estimated that 27 million Americans have some form of thyroid disease and about ½ are undiagnosed. Women outnumber men in incidence, with 8 of 10 thyroid patients being female. Women are estimated to be 5 to 8 times more likely than men to have *hypo*thyroidism. Of the two types of malfunction of the thyroid, hypothyroidism is more common.

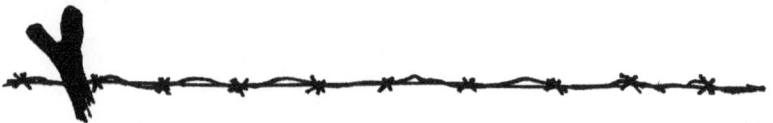

And its symptoms are more likely to be self-diagnosed as age or mileage.

The function of the thyroid gland is to produce thyroid hormone, a substance that is absolutely vital. In the developing child, it affects growth and development including brain function. It's so vital that all states have now enacted requirements for screening of newborns for inborn hypothyroidism. Detection and treatment of a lack of thyroid in the infant prevents a form of mental retardation. But not all hypothyroidism is inborn and evident at birth. Most of it occurs in adults. The prevalence increases after the age of 35 and it is high in women over age 50.

Even though we're no longer growing, thyroid hormone is still vital for adults. Adequate levels of the hormone are required for basic metabolism, particularly the usage of fat and carbohydrates; heart function; basic chemical function of all cells; muscle tone and strength; and absorption of nutrients from the intestines. Thyroid hormone levels affect mood, personality, ability to think, and sleep patterns and affect the function of other glands, particularly the reproductive system.

The most common cause of hypothyroidism is autoimmune—the body attacks itself. In this case, the attack is on the thyroid. It's not clear exactly why this happens. Other causes of hypothyroidism are: treatment of *hyper*thyroidism by destruction of the gland using radiation, chemicals or surgery; inability to produce thyroid hormone because of cellular defects in the gland or because of an iodine deficiency; medications such as lithium or amiodarone; or other autoimmune diseases such as scleroderma.

Why would such an important disease be mistaken as "just aging" or wearing out? The answer is that because of the thyroid's normal function, a reduction in that function makes it seem that everything is slowing down. No acute pain, no dramatic symptoms, just slower and slower function. If it's not corrected and there's essentially *no* thyroid function the result can be coma and death. But the slow decline is seen

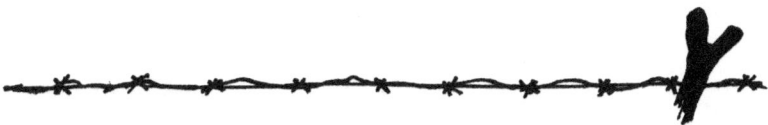

as a series of vague, almost indefinable problems. The include: weight gain, depressed mood, fatigue, sleepiness, intolerance to cold, lowered body temperature, puffy eyes, weakness, muscle aches and joint complaints. Also noted are problems with balance, dry skin, thinning hair, loss of body hair and some eyebrows, sallow skin, slowed heartbeat, constipation, and "looking older." I could continue with even more signs, but you get the point.

Once discovered, hypothyroidism is easy to treat with daily medication. But, to diagnose it, your health care provider must do a lab test. This test is recommended by the American Thyroid Association as screening at five year intervals for all over age 35. It's particularly important for women over 50. Even so, some health care providers don't include this in regular screening, particularly if the patient doesn't complain of any of the symptoms. At your next regular health exam, ask if you've been screened for thyroid disease. Remember, it's up to you to mention these vague problems if you experience them. Each sign or symptom could be caused by other health conditions, but they can also signal a reduction in thyroid function.

—Teddy

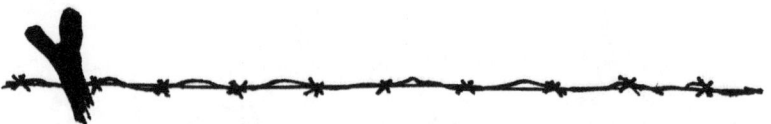

Capsule 55

Baling Wire, Duct Tape And Other Handy Stuff

A bale of hay held together by wire is an uncommon sight these days. Twine or a wider bale wrapper made of plastic is now more often used to assemble hay. But that doesn't mean that baling wire is no longer useful. As any farm or ranch person knows, baling wire's flexibility and strength combine to make it the perfect item for a multitude of temporary repairs. Lose a bolt? Muffler sagging? Hole in the fence? Just bring out the baling wire.

Another item of many uses is duct tape. It's not just useful for covering a tear in the pickup seat cover. Applied with care and in liberal amounts, it can become a "spot weld" on a rusty grain truck bed, saving precious wheat enroute to the elevator. Or, a neat little wad of it covered by several strong wraps of same can repair a pellet gun's damage to plastic irrigation pipe.

If you're prone to improvise, you will be able to construct a shade shelter for a small animal or the frame for a compost pile from the pallets that the seed sacks arrived on. In fact, you can probably make a long list of the ways you have taken an item intended for one use and created another purpose for it. Making that list could be an interesting coffee shop discussion topic.

Before you start making your list, let me tell you about an alternate use for monofilament fishing line. If you are a diabetic, or know someone

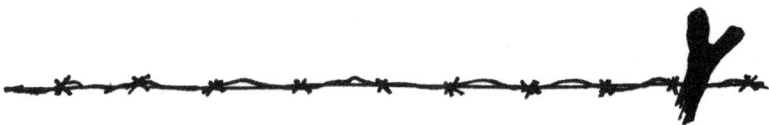

who is, this can be important for you. Since there are 15.7 million diabetics in the U.S., with about 798,000 new cases diagnosed each year, chances are that you know someone to whom this could be helpful.

Some background information will make the explanation clearer. As you know, diabetes is diagnosed when the body cannot properly use the glucose (sugar) that we all need for proper body function. Either there is not enough insulin produced by the pancreas or the body is resistant to the insulin present and cannot utilize it properly, or a combination of those two problems. Depending on the type of diabetes, a person may need to take oral medication, insulin, or a combination. Besides medication, diet and exercise prescriptions are provided to attempt to keep the blood glucose level within normal limits. If the blood glucose is not well controlled, several complications can occur. One of those is poor circulation due to malfunction in the small blood vessels. This poor circulation can affect the eyes, the kidneys, and often affects the hands and feet. Another complication is neuropathy (nerve damage) particularly in the feet and hands.

If the person has even the smallest injury to the foot, reduced sensation caused by the nerve damage may allow a splinter or blister or small skin infection to go unnoticed. The poor circulation makes healing slow or ineffective. One dreaded result is gangrene and the need for amputation.

Now, here's where that monofilament fishing line come in. A little tool, called the Semmes-Weinstein monofilament, which resembles a toothbrush with a single bristle (about two inches of that fishing line) is used to test the sensation of several spots on each foot. Using a diagram to note the results, the spots are touched just firmly enough to make the filament bend slightly. Loss of or reduced sensation is an indication of developing neuropathy. The recommendation is that at least once each year, the health care provider do this screening test for each diabetic in order to be aware of any changes or developing problems. It's such a

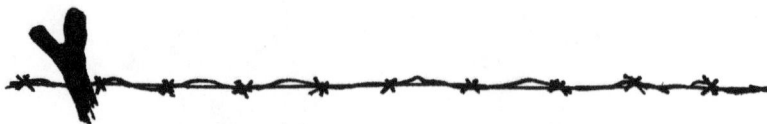

good idea that the government will send a patient their own little fishing line apparatus to use at home. Just go to the Internet Web Site www.bphc.hrsa.gov/leap to request the tool and educational materials.

This screening is only one part of good care for diabetes, but it is an important part. If you know a diabetic, encourage that person to ask their health care provider about doing the screening, if it is not regularly part of the care they receive. And tell them how to get their own little "fishing line" tool. They won't catch a trout on it, but they might prevent an amputation.

—Teddy

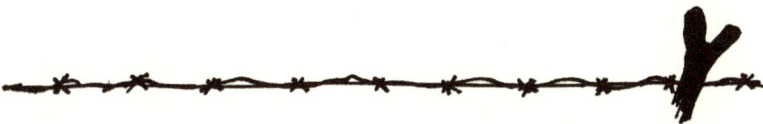

Capsule 56

Avoiding The Shrink

I've moved my base of covert operation to the Dairy Queen. Now, don't let that lead you to think that I've gone completely off the edge and that the title of this refers to staying away from psychiatrists.

I haven't begun to suspect conspiracies or to plot survival strategies. The covert operation I'm talking about is my "incidental listening." Some might call it eavesdropping. Regardless, my hearing is pretty good and I hear more at the DQ than at the post office (my other main stop when I go into town). Conversations at the post office tend to be short. And since my "listening" is selective, picking up only items relating to health, the new site has more to offer.

"If I had been a feeder calf, we'd have lost money on me because of the shrink they put me on before that surgery," Charlie, a local rancher said from the booth in front of mine. Surgery. Careful to look only into my coffee cup, I tuned right in and waited to hear about the "shrink."

What he was referring to was the typical weight loss that occurs in cattle during the process of moving from pasture to feedlot or to market due to lack of food and water and the effect of the stress of transport on the bowels and kidneys. Those cattle shrink.

Charlie made a pretty good case for the possibility that he'd shrunk also. He had surgery in a town seventy miles from home. Instructions were to be at the hospital the morning of surgery at 6:30 a.m., for a

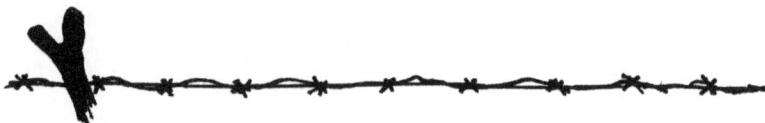

procedure at 10:00 a.m. The last thing he was told was, "Nothing by mouth after midnight."

Accustomed to an early bedtime and knowing he had to be up early to get on the road, Charlie went to bed about 8:00 p.m. By the time his operation actually began, at 2:00 p.m. (rescheduled, unavoidable, they told him), Charlie had been without food or fluids for 18 hours. No wonder he was feeling as if he had shrunk.

According to research reported in the *American Journal of Nursing*, Charlie's experience is not uncommon. Beyond that, in most cases it is not necessary.

Many years ago, the routine of fasting after midnight prior to surgery developed because it was thought that an empty stomach would reduce the hazard of pneumonia caused by inhalation of stomach contents. Vomiting after and sometimes during anesthesia was common in those days. Anesthesia has improved and nausea and vomiting are no longer the rule with surgery. Studies have shown that there is little scientific evidence to support the lengthy fasting requirements. So, in an attempt to improve practice and to improve comfort for patients, the American Society of Anesthesiologists issued guidelines for preoperative fasting in 1999. Those guidelines state that for healthy patients undergoing elective surgery (not women in labor or emergency surgery patients):

- ✪ Clear liquids can be allowed up to 2 hours before surgery. Clear liquids are water, fruit juice without pulp, carbonated beverages, clear tea, and black coffee.
- ✪ A light meal can be allowed up to six hours before surgery. A light meal would be dry toast and clear liquids, no fatty foods, no meat.

So, according to those guidelines, Charlie could have had his morning coffee. Perhaps that would have prevented a caffeine withdrawal headache. He could have had water to reduce thirst and prevent dehydration. He could have had fruit juice to stave off low blood sugar.

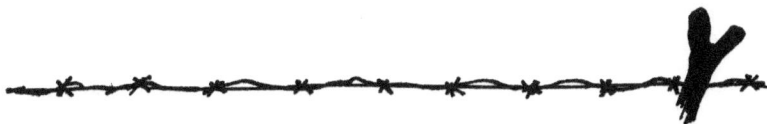

If the surgery was rescheduled as much as six hours in advance, he could have had the light meal. Chicken bouillon, cherry gelatin and dry toast might have looked good by then.

Why was he "shrunk?" The research I mentioned earlier, conducted at a large hospital in Dallas, showed that the 155 patients surveyed had fasted for an average of 12 hours, some fasting as long as 20 hours from liquids and 37 hours from solids. Ninety-seven percent had no liquids for more than six hours. Apparently, even though the guidelines were published in 1999, it is taking a while for practice to catch up.

Aside for feeling some sympathy for Charlie and others who follow the old "nothing by mouth after midnight" routine, what can a person do? As with most things related to your health care, you can speak up when it affects you or your family. If you are told "nothing by mouth after midnight," ask why. If the response is not satisfactory, mention the guidelines from the American Society of Anesthesiologists. Those are available on the Internet at the following website www.asahq.org/practice/npo/npoguide.html.

If you are still not getting anywhere, request to speak to the anesthesiologist or your surgeon. Ask whether you are a person to whom the guidelines apply. How else can you get your morning coffee or tea or avoid the shrink?

—Teddy

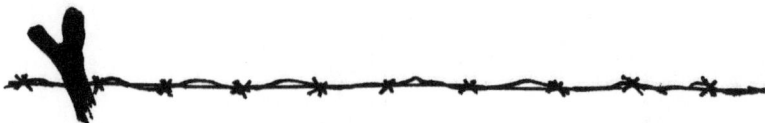

Capsule 57

Don't Miss The Point

*H*ave you ever listened to a story or a joke and at the end been left wondering, "What was the point?" That has probably happened to each of us sometime. We do get the point though, when there is something in the story that makes it real or important for us.

Here's an example. A friend who works with cattle was telling me about a sick calf he had. The first signs of illness were pretty general. The animal was off his feed, was isolating himself and was down a lot. It had not been too many days since the calf had been transformed into a steer, so his wound was not completely healed. Our cattleman friend said that the next day the young steer's eyes had begun to "roll back" and he was sicker, had fever. His prediction was an imminent death preceded by muscle rigidity and backward arching of the back. The image that suggested was not pretty.

It's not idle curiosity that caused my interest. It's a nurse thing. We have to know. "What do you think is wrong?" I asked. "My guess is tetanus," he said. Now he really had my attention. I was getting a point.

Immunization for tetanus, among several other diseases is a routine part of well-child care. In fact, it has become so routine that it is easy to forget the reasons for the immunizations. Few of us have ever seen tetanus in humans. In developed countries where immunizations are mandatory for children, the incidence of many diseases has dropped

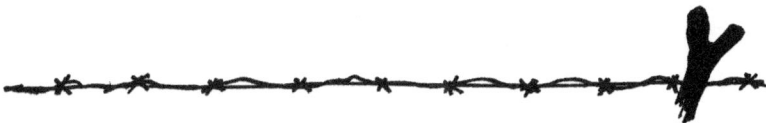

dramatically. Tetanus is among those. Childhood immunization in the U.S. has reduced to a small number (less than 70) the annually reported cases of tetanus. About 95% of those cases are in persons 20 years of age or older. Deaths do still occur in greater numbers in undeveloped countries or where immunization is not routine.

People who work on farms or ranches are particularly at risk to encounter tetanus because of the way the organism that causes it lives naturally. Clostridium tetani is present normally (not causing disease) in the intestinal tract of horses, cattle, and humans. Untreated feces deposits the organism in the soil. It dries as a spore and can be carried in dust. When the organism enters a wound that is closed to the air, the tetani begin to grow and form a toxin. The toxin is the poison that causes the illness. That steer probably got contaminated dirt in his castration wound.

Fortunately for us humans, the vaccine will help us make antibodies that will prevent the disease. But, one immunization is not enough. An initial series of three shots is needed. This series is part of the required childhood vaccination nowadays. For children, the tetanus is combined with diphtheria and pertussis (whooping cough) as one dose. If you were ever in the military, you were sure to get the series there. But, some older people or those from some foreign countries may not have had the full series.

After the original series, to keep immunity at the right level, boosters are required. The Advisory Committee on Immunization Practice recommends a booster every 10 years for all adults who had an initial series. If a person has an injury that is contaminated with dirt, feces, saliva, or is a burn or puncture wound or frostbite and it has been more than 5 years since the booster, an additional booster should be given. For clean, minor wounds with the ten-year period, no booster is required.

The alternative to an adequate series of vaccinations (original 3 plus boosters) is the use of tetanus antitoxin in situations with potentially

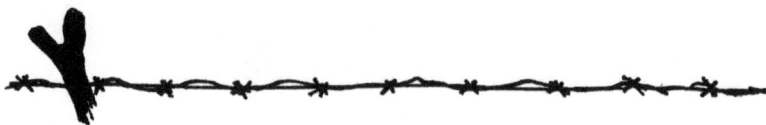

contaminated wounds. This is not an attractive option because there are risks of serious reactions to the antitoxins.

It's a simple thing to get a booster. And it's an important thing to have both the basic series and the regular boosters. But, it's also easy to forget until it is too late. One way to avoid forgetting is to do the following: (1) decide today to check the immunization status of each person in your family and of each person who works for you, (2) if anyone has no record of their immunization, start one today and put it in a safe place, and (3) if anyone is lacking the basic series for tetanus, take them to the local clinic or health department to start the series. For adults the primary series is two doses given at least four weeks apart and the third dose is given 6–12 months after the second. If the history is uncertain, a person should receive the full series. Resolve to have your booster every ten years. Remember, any costs for the time and effort to do this are far less than the potential cost of treating the serious illness that a case of human tetanus would bring.

That's a long story starting with a sick steer. Now that I have told it to you, my question is this. Do you get the point—the needle point?

—Teddy

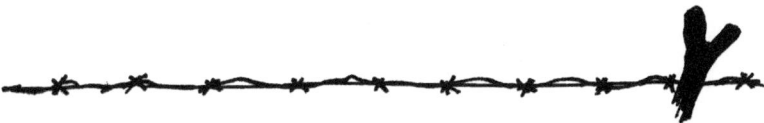

Capsule 58

Immunization for Heartache

*T*he inevitable happened at our house a couple of weeks ago. One of my teenage daughters had her heart broken by a young man she really liked.

Fortunately for her, I have had my heart broken numerous times. I say fortunately because who better to commiserate with than someone who knows that a heartache crushes the spirit. The writer of Proverbs even used that phrase.

For two or three days, my baby had the characteristic loss of appetite, listless spirit, and that look in her eyes. She cried, she slept a lot, she wrote in her journal, and then she came to me.

I rubbed her back and played with her hair and said nothing. I knew that when she was ready to talk, we would. And, we eventually did, lying side by side on my bed. We hashed it out, this tale of first love lost, knowing that nothing was going to change the circumstances despite our best efforts to recall the past.

Hurt is hurt and sometimes a person just has to hurt it out.

Predictably, she soon was on the mend. Our talks turned to more mundane matters like Spanish tests that were "sooooooooo hard." She even began to laugh again at my ability to misplace things and then remember in the middle of the night where they were.

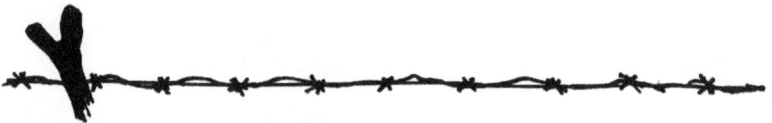

I wondered if I should tell her what lies ahead. That heartaches of this life are only beginning and that her mother won't always be around to comfort her the way I was this time.

Somehow I think she already knows that. Most of us have it figured out before we're twenty that life is going to throw at us far more than we can catch.

Heartache at 16 or 66 may carry a different perspective, but the impact is the same. Our desire to be comforted during such times remains an instinctive need.

My mother used to tell me that she wished she had a magic wand to wave to make the hurt go away. She also taught me about a natural immunization that worked for us as children. Band-aids, cookies, and hugs went a long way not just for scraped knees but for hurt feelings. You don't have to have an HMO for those.

When the inevitable heartache happens to someone you love or even to you, treat it with some of the proverbial tender, loving care. It's a prescription that can be filled anywhere, anytime.

—Sue Jane

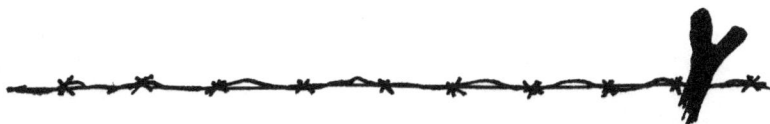

Capsule 59

My Home Sweet Home

Road trips.

Those two words may rekindle the worst of memories for some folks but not for me. Road trips and I were meant for each other. I never got car-sick, I hated to fly, and even as a child I was precociously in awe of my surroundings.

The love of travel was nurtured by parents who piled their five children in the family station wagon and took off to visit family or friends in Washington state, Virginia, and Alabama. That last one was a doozy-the oldest of my siblings was 12 and the youngest 10 months old. And for some strange reason, my dad decided to rent a trailer and pull it along, too. Yes, we camped out, and miraculously my mother lived to tell about it.

My two daughters and I have kept the family tradition, except for the trailer trip. I taught them to repeat after me, "Hotels are our friends."

To the great Northwest to the East Coast throughout the Deep South and all over our great state of Texas, my girls and I have experienced firsthand why the United States is a land to love. Its geography is as varied as the people who inhabit it, and it is important for me as a parent for my children to appreciate the variety.

Our rural home is secluded, a county with only one town and

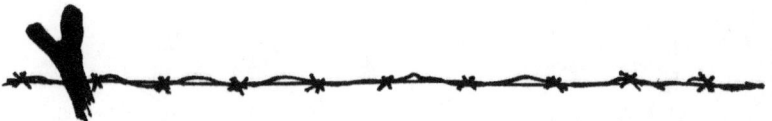

one school. It is a haven for education, for peace and quiet, and for raising children in what is pretty much a safe place.

Nothing stifles growth, however, more than a smugness as well as a naiveté that one's own little world is the only world that exists. That is especially true if that little world is, by most accounts, safe and secure.

Those girls have seen the swells of the oceans on both coasts, each time venturing out a little farther than they did the first time they experienced it. They have taken nervous and then excited glances over the edge of mountain roads that were a far cry from their flat farm-to-market roads back home. And they have learned that it is o.k. to buy a rose from or give money to a street person.

Travel has taught lessons I could not, and road trips in particular gave the three of us time alone in the car with the view, a good book, the license plate game, and plenty of good music. They have suffered through my CDs of Merle Haggard, but they have learned to love James Taylor as much as their mother does.

What remarkable treasures we have in the United States, basically "free" for the taking. Make a few cuts in family entertainment throughout the year, and then take a road trip at some point. This land was made for you and me. Take it as needed, but often.

—Sue Jane

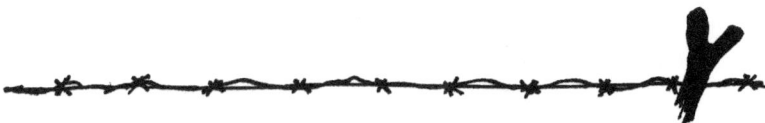

Capsule 60

Blame It on the Weather

Geographical enabling. I think I will coin that phrase and see if I can gain some notoriety in a psychology textbook.

The theory goes something like this: obsessive-compulsive behavior appears in a high rate of West Texas women (and other farm and ranch women) because of the weather indigenous to their area. Sounds intellectually shallow, doesn't it?

However, I believe I am on to something here, especially since I admit now to the world and myself that I, too, have that obsessive-compulsive tendency in my behavior. (What is it with hyphenated words in psycho-babble jargon?)

Think about it. In West Texas, as in most of the farming and ranching country, our weather is unpredictable and often extreme. When it's hot, it's really hot. If it rains, it is going to rain and rain and rain. If it isn't going to rain, we have droughts. Long ones that kill your grass before you can even grow it. And of course there's the wind—breezes do not exist in West Texas. It's probably the same where you live. Breezes are for sissy parts of the country. It blows hard out here or it doesn't blow at all.

Because I am but a product of my environment, I can't help but do things in the extreme. If I make homemade ice cream, I think I must eat it all—in one evening. All four quarts. If I clean house, I must do it

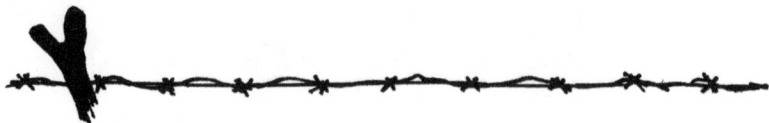

all—between 11:30 p.m. to 2 a.m. That's because from 6 p.m. to 11:30 p.m. I had to take a nap to rest.

And credit card companies love people from farm and ranch areas like West Texas. If we shop, we do it all at once. Impulsive spending. Borrow-my-sister's-van-kind-of-spending so I'll have more room for all the sacks.

There's no such thing as going to the grocery store and buying one thing—I live in the country and feel like I must buy four loaves of bread, a case of toilet paper, and six-months supply of dishwashing detergent. This is especially pitiful because I don't even cook to get dishes dirty. Sadly, my storage building is full of contact lens solution. I wear glasses but it was too good a buy to turn down.

The only way to solve my problem is to pay big bucks for a therapist or move to a place where the weather stays the same year round so I can settle into some equilibrium—like a tropical climate. Costa Rica? The Bahamas? Cancún? I'm also bad at making decisions. I wonder who or what I can blame *that* on.

—Sue Jane

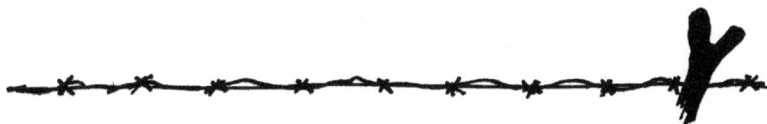

Capsule 61

Aunt Bert

My mother's middle sister was a farm girl from Fisher County, Texas, whose life mirrored the tough times of the Depression era in which she grew up. Roberta Clark's spirit reflected the strength of the people who survived that time.

Recognizing my voice when I would call, Aunt Bert would say in a perky, petite voice, "Well, hello my dear." It was a chipper but sincere voice. The last time I heard it, the chipper part was missing. She passed away that same night in 2003, just a few hours after our last phone conversation. The inevitable memories have flowed since that time, wonderful memories of an aunt beloved for so many reasons.

She was the quintessential "cool" aunt. There was an element of mystery for she was also the aunt who lived far away, wrote letters sealed in air mail envelopes, and sent those birthday cards with the money slots full of dimes.

In addition, Aunt Bert was the queen of style. Not the trendy fashion, but the classic look. My sister recalled the time our aunt showed up one summer in this sleek, sleeveless red dress and high heels. We recall her standing in the doorway, looking svelte and suave, smoking her long-tipped cigarette. If anyone could glamorize a dreaded vice, it was Aunt Bert. During her smoking years, her voice was raspy but her smell was sweet. She exuded an aroma of tenderness as she would hold

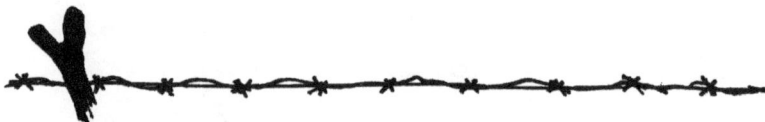

us close, reading to us, or telling us a story about how mischievous our mother was as a little girl.

One time she paid me a half dollar to sit still so Mother could brush my hair. She was either really rich, I thought, or I was acting very, very badly.

Those were my childhood recollections. It was not until years later that I learned those years were very painful ones for her personally. Two marriages had failed with physical abuse involved in one. There would also be a self-imposed distance from her Texas roots that geographically she would never reconcile. But even with her personal pain and turmoil, she took the time and effort to be a special aunt.

When I was five, Aunt Bert married again. Uncle Peter was a keeper, this Long Island New Yorker. He was the man who made my aunt laugh again. I grew to love him for that simple fact. It took him a while to adjust to having a sister-in-law with five children, but he eventually warmed to the fact that kids were kids. Once he sent me a reel for my fishing rod because he knew I liked to fish as he did. Uncle Peter and Aunt Bert also answered my letters, which made me eager to write more.

My aunt had two passions outside of family. Her first one was her love for her pets. When we were sending her our school pictures, she would mail us photos of George Albert or Charlie Brown, her Siamese cats. Then came the Airedales: Sky, Pete, Amber, Aran, and Shandy. Morgan leFay, a wire-haired terrier, thought by many to be Uncle Peter reincarnated, would be with her the night she died.

The other joy came from her garden. It was no doubt her connection to her widowed mother, my grandmother, who had found much solace in tending her own flowers on dry Texas farmland until her death in 1955. Aunt Bert's garden was at her home on Washington state's Olympic Peninsula, but a garden is a garden anywhere when it's tended with love. Aunt Bert knew how to do that. The view from her backyard

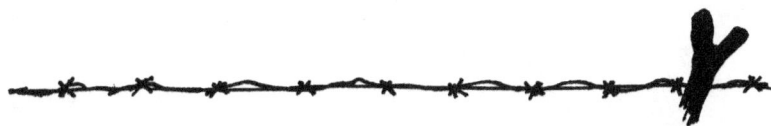

deck overlooking her flowers and the bay was postcard material.

When my daughters were born, Aunt Bert gifted them with Christmas stockings, handmade treasures done to perfection in needlepoint. She also made a quilt for my younger daughter, Emily. Through the years, she nurtured the relationship with her great-nieces as well, answering all the letters they wrote to her. Both girls have inherited their great-aunt's love for animals. And this spring my older daughter will come home to plant my flowerbeds, something she has done for years, part of Aunt Bert's legacy, I think. They have also learned that the best hand-me-downs are family traditions, and Aunt Bert helped them learn that lesson.

I have an original 1957 edition of *How the Grinch Stole Christmas*. Written inside the front cover is "To Susie, Merry Christmas to my buddy, from Auntie Bert." From now on at Christmas, when the girls hang the stockings she made and I get out the keepsake book, we will be blessed to remember the bond we had with her, a special memory bouquet that isn't seasonal but endures like the perennials she grew in her garden.

—Sue Jane

 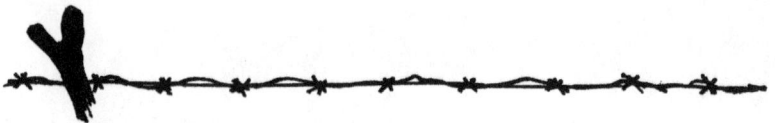

Capsule 62

Stay-at-Home Dad

*H*oward Espy ranched.

For someone like me who wouldn't know much about the particulars of that job, his daughter Mary John clued me in one afternoon as we talked about her childhood in Sutton County near Sonora, Texas, in the 1950s.

Ranching for Mr. Espy meant milking cows, shearing sheep, and doctoring all the livestock from the dreaded screwworm. He did it meticulously, carefully, and often with Mary John, whom he called Little Bit, right by his side. Mary John, herself now a rancher's wife on a farm in Borden County where I live, explained to me that her father was a master at using such moments to teach his young daughters.

Holding sheep during shearing time "was an honor" because working beside Dad was the ultimate bond of trust. He knew his daughters had been attentive and could do the work they had seen him perform so many times before.

Daily doctoring of the goats, sheep, and cattle was the norm in the 1950s because the screwworm eradication program had not yet begun. To be negligent at this particular ranching chore might mean the loss of an entire herd. It would be Mary John's favorite ranching chore, the doctoring of those animals. I like to imagine the security her father's tender care of his animals must have given to this child. If Dad loves

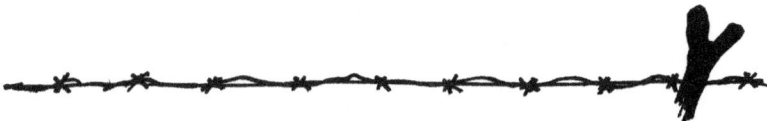

these animals enough to watch over them so diligently, I know he's going to do the same and more for me, might think Little Bit.

She was right. With tenderness, Mr. Espy placed Little Bit as a toddler on a pillow in front of him while on a "good ol' sorrel mare." This was how she learned to ride. With caution, he did not allow his daughters to wear a belt while riding or to carry a rope in order to prevent getting hung up.

Having a stay-at-home Dad had other benefits. His love of cooking brought him in for the big noon meal early to help Mrs. Espy. Dad made the homemade biscuits. Little Bit learned to eat some of the finer things in life as her dad mixed butter and Brer Rabbit syrup to smooth over those biscuits.

When Dad had checked his last animal and checked the gates to close out a day's work, his evening wasn't spent in a recliner in front of the television. He didn't insist on "his time" to rest by himself without distraction of little feet running around him. He sat on the front porch and watched the clouds in anticipation of rain, and Little Bit sat with him. Sutton County in the 1950s was in the midst of an eight-year drought, so evenings on the porch might not produce the desired weather-related results. Mr. Espy, however, was soaking in precious time with his daughter.

Those experiences remain vivid for my friend: the tastes of cold water on a hot day, of a sweet cookie dipped in stout Cowboy coffee, of dust on the trail of a 25-mile cattle drive to town she got to make one time with her dad. Too soon her experiences became memories as Mr. Espy died when Mary John was only 13.

The unpretentious man who would come home and take his spurs off before going to town to get something for the ranch ("no need wearing them if they aren't in use") was a provider in the classic sense of the word. Whether a man lives to a ripe old age or dies young becomes a non-issue when he lives the way Mr. Espy did. He gave Little Bit a whole lot of memories.

—Sue Jane

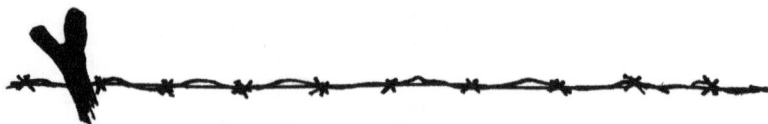

Capsule 63

Collateral

A lock box is magic in the hands of a grandchild, even if that grandchild is 48 years old. As my mother emptied the contents of her mother's rusted metal container, it was like watching a rabbit pulled from a hat. But the animals that emerged weren't rabbits, they turned out to be four mules, their story contained on a single piece of paper in grandmother's old documents.

There were four mules on my grandmother's farm: Jack, John, Jude, and Old Red. The fact that she named them makes me think she valued them for more than just plow and pack animals. In 1936, mules were worked hard; in January of that year, they added another notch to their resumé. They became collateral.

The original bank note, now in my mother's possession, tells a story familiar to farmers of that decade. Taxes were due at the end of January; that total came to $163 for the 220 acres my widowed grandmother farmed and used as pasture. The date on the term note is January, 1936. It was due as soon as the cotton was harvested.

The value as seen typed on the note for the mules was listed at $500.00. A description of the four animals indicated that three were young and one was soft-mouthed—probably Old Red. Also included was their height—perhaps the bankers loaned more money on tall mules.

At the bottom of the note is a stamp marked paid, dated November

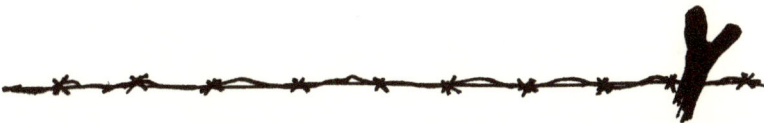

1, 1936. Old Red, Jack, John, and Jude did not have to be sacrificed for the sake of the land. The debt was paid, and no evidence exists that she ever had to use them again in that way.

From January to November of that year, Grandmother probably had some tense moments. She must have wondered if the mules would stay healthy. Were the rains going to come? I also can imagine some restless nights when thunderstorms could bring needed rain but dreaded hail.

Reading over this old document gave me some glimpse at my grandmother's character. The farm was fiercely important to her, her word was good, and her work ethic even better.

From 1931 on, there was no husband or soulmate to help my grandmother with difficult decisions such as paying taxes, but she had four mules who were good for a $163 note.

I'm sure she considered them priceless.

—Sue Jane

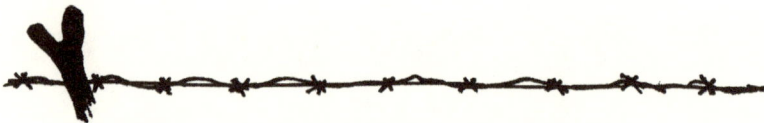

Capsule 64

Coming Home

*A*h, the one-horse town. Great for raising kids, peace and quiet, and avoiding rush hour traffic jams.

Angst for teenagers who long for a Sonic Drive-In around the corner instead of 30 miles down the road.

I honestly think the teenagers in our town have a ceremony, raise their right hands, and swear on a Bible held by the class president. The oath is, "I, (state your name), will never, ever come back to Small Town, America."

Throughout college, my older daughter honored that oath. She seldom returned for the Friday night football games, avoided homecoming festivities, and worked her summers in her college town. She meant what she said, and she said what she meant.

Then it happened—early July in the summer she was to graduate from college.

Most people do enjoy going to town on the Fourth simply because of the fireworks display. Booths vending various wares and carnivals are a draw, too, but the grand finale in the sky is what it's all about. We had always driven the thirty minutes to the next town to watch the pinwheels and rockets with family and friends.

But on this occasion, Julie wanted to come home. Home didn't have fireworks. Home didn't have booths, and the closest thing to a

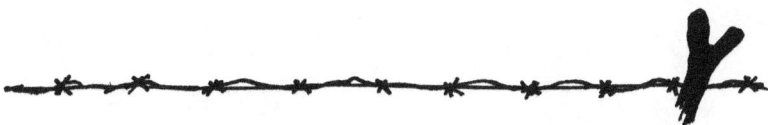

carnival ride I could offer would be a spin on the neighbor's golf cart.

What home did have, and what Julie had grown to miss, was the very thing she swore off years earlier. She had grown to miss nothing to do.

College years were spent studying and working, of course, but with the added attractions of dancing, going to movies, eating out, and late-night coffee shop runs. And she loved it. But, she also knew that now there was something to be said for nothing.

Nothing means watching old home movies because there aren't any theaters. Nothing means making homemade ice cream because there's no Dairy Queen in sight. Nothing means brewing up some coffee and sitting on the couch to talk to your mother about anything except what's going to be on a test.

It took a while, but my daughter finally came home.

At some point, it's what many rural native sons and daughters do. Searches for meaningful work, greater flexibility in schedules, social opportunities often take them away from their rural settings. Then, a funny thing happens on the way to the bank. They realize that meaningful work might just be found in the one county library or the lone post office or the rural school.

They come to understand that farmers and ranchers are quite familiar with flexibility because the elements directly affect their daily chore list. They must be flexible and their work must reflect that.
And as for social opportunity, the small town creates its own with fall festivals, impromptu neighborhood barbecues, and high school athletic events catered by concession stands selling homemade items.

"Coming home" may not be a permanent move—my daughter has no plans to settle here, at least for now. The concept involves something far more important. Coming home is about appreciating the slower, simpler life that is often equated with country living.

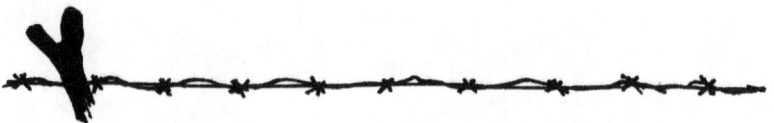

Someday when my daughter is sitting behind that desk in an office in Manhattan or Boston or Seattle, she will find herself able to come home any time. She can catch the next flight and be there physically. Or she can sit back, close her eyes, and appreciate the memories of a childhood spent in a small town in West Texas.

—Sue Jane

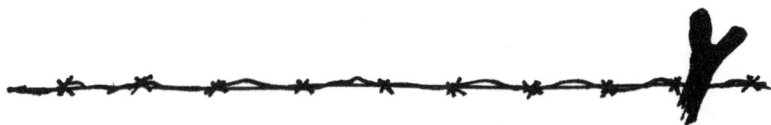

Capsule 65

Investing in Order to Preserve

*D*espite a lifetime of acquaintance, there's still quite a bit I don't know about Billie and Bobby McCormick. I don't know much about their childhoods, their high school years, the story of their courtship and marriage, or even their favorite things. I do know that Bobby grew up in Snyder, Texas, in a large family, Billie graduated with honors from Abilene High School, they met at college, married and came back to Snyder where Bobby worked in the family business while Billie stayed home and had a business of her own, called "Mom's In the House."

They were friends of my mom and dad. They shared similar life and family circumstances. There was the college connection, the church connection, the-having-children-about-the-same-age connection, the progressive dinners connection, etc.

They are still my parents' friends. Even though their circumstances are no longer the same, the sentimental bond and the memories remain. More importantly, Bobby and Billie are now *my* friends. I'm near the half-century mark, and Bobby and Billie have always been around. Their physical bodies are worn from numerous surgeries and from Parkinson's Disease, but their spiritual health is not in question—it only grows stronger.

I see this spiritual growth in many of my parents' friends from

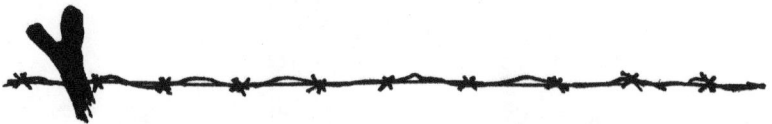

my early years. And those early years for me were the 1960s and 1970s—an unsettling time in a country at war with others and itself.

It was not easy to rear children in the 60s and 70s. Responsibilities of parenthood never are a snap, but parents then had to contend with such an enormous social upheaval. The dilemmas of long hair, draft dodging, bucking the establishment, the sexual openness of the era were tough calls for a generation reared in the dutiful 1940s. My parents and their friends were torn between following their parental instincts and the rigid religious and social expectations of the day.

Lifetime friendships produced the inevitable—the sharing of the good, the bad, and the ugly. The bad and the ugly usually came from personality conflicts, philosophical differences, and preferences on how things were to be done. How nice to have mentors who survived what were difficult times, learned from those moments, and today share their love for each other and their wisdom with me. That's the good part.

Examples of kinship like this one, which is essentially a cycle of love, exist in abundance for farm and ranch families. Because generations of families often dwell on property bordering other generations of families, a rural neighborhood may see little turnover. People grow up knowing each other's family histories in addition to their own.

Rather than a Hatfield and McCoy scenario, country neighbors know their reliance and trust on each other is vital. There are farm animals, crops, and implements that require daily attention. When a disability comes, rural friends have to be there for each other. When a vacation is needed, country neighbors take on extra work to give time for their neighbors' getaway. Both family and friends invest in the one another in direct physical assistance and emotional concern.

Twenty years ago, I moved away from the town where Bobby and Billie still live. I am their rural neighbor. Though 30 miles down the road, we are here (and there) for each other. They still drive out to our

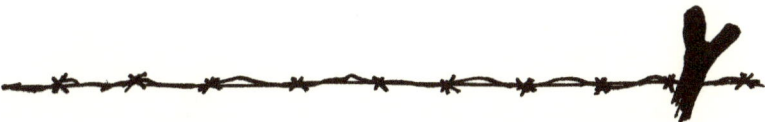

small town to watch my children play ball. I see them when I drive in to their town for church.

The formula for preserving and nurturing both friendships and farms/ranches is the same. Invest some time and energy in the lives of the people around you. The harvest will be plentiful.

—Sue Jane

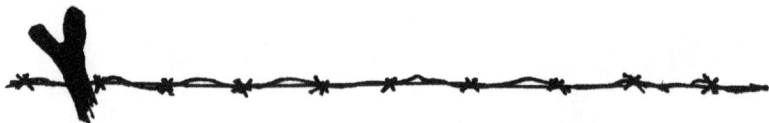

Capsule 66

Getting In Touch With The Feminine Side

Growing up a bona fide tomboy, I placed no priority on nurturing relationships with girls. Girls gossiped, they did not know how to throw a baseball, and they worried far too much about their hair. And whoever wanted to spend time decorating her face was stupid—that's what coloring books were for. I liked those smelly boys because they picked me first to be on their teams. We shared our baseball cards and if I decided to renege on a trade, it was no big deal—we worked it out without tears or cross words.

My preference for male social company continues to this day. Baseball cards go a long way in building a rapport with the male students in my English classes. Once they find out I like baseball, I sense a little bit more respect comes my way.

I still hate purses and putting on make-up, but in my 40s I've made great strides with getting in touch with my feminine self.

This remarkable (according to my sisters) feat has been accomplished by a proactive stance I began a few years ago when I planned a girls' night out for some women with whom I worked.

One of our own had finished her chemotherapy for a brain tumor and a few of us thought it would be fun to take her to Lubbock for something other than a doctor visit. We went to see a movie and subsequently started the tradition that whatever letter the title of the

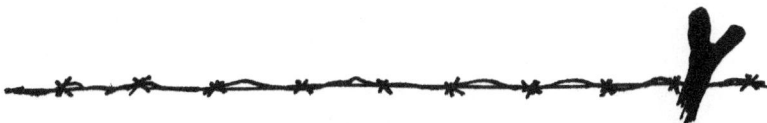

movie began with, we had to eat at a restaurant with that same first letter. Our first date was watching "Zorro" and eating at a restaurant named Zucchini's. Not bad for our first trip.

Our friend died less than two years later, but not before we made three more outings. Her daughter-in-law has since moved to our community and has joined in our times together. The movie trips are not as frequent as we would like, but the times together go a long way in reviving our sense of sisterhood as we talk about spouses, kids, and what diet we are on. Heavier topics are for other times. This is just for fun and just for women.

Besides my colleagues, I enjoy a biological sisterhood with two younger sisters and two cousins—all school teachers. Our "sorority" specializes in taking exciting journeys. Our trips have included a cross-country trip in a 1984 Ford truck. If the trip had been in 1984, that would have been fine, but it was in the summer of '96 and the air conditioner went out.

In the summer of '97 we wanted to tour the antebellum homes in Louisiana and Mississippi. Actually, what we did was to also tour as many fine dining establishments—and there are plenty in the South from which to choose. We came home with the traditional souvenirs—bigger thighs and tighter clothes.

Before this last trip to Manzanita, Oregon, I got a manicure, pedicure, and had my hair done. The only lapse from the feminine that I had the entire trip was wanting to throw the football on the beach. But, I did make sure that I didn't break a nail.

It's especially crucial for women who live in the country to discover that feminine side. Their chores often require getting dirty nails and even dirtier boots. Their company is often mostly male. Gender lines have a tendency to blur if women don't take the initiative.

Most successful and peaceful rural women I know have learned the secret to finding and flaunting their femininity. They take baths, usually

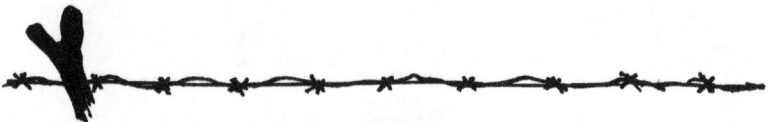

four-hour bubble baths. Showers are for cleaning, but baths do the trick when a woman just needs to relax and feel like a woman.

If a man built your house and you don't have a bath, just use a horse trough. Lather up and soak—if it's outside the barn, you'll get a good tan.

Then after that long bath, get in the ol' pick-up truck, drive on down the road, pick up the gals, and head out for a movie or a meal or a dance without the guys.

I say leave them home and let them clean the tub. It will help them get in touch with *their* feminine side.

—Sue Jane

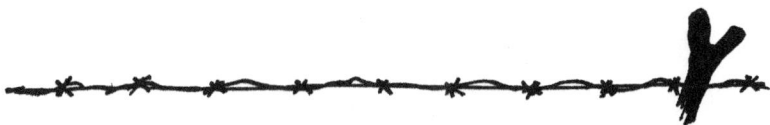

Capsule 67

Why I Love October And Baseball...And Hate Snakes

*I*n the small town where we grew up, Scotty and I dug holes in the front yard and used Dad's driver and three wood to putt. We practiced Punt, Pass, and Kick out in the road. We ran races that I never won. And, we played sandlot baseball. I did not walk in my brother's shadow. I was his shadow.

For much of our childhood in the late 50s and early 60s, we roamed during our afternoons after school and most of our summer days. Though the two of us had each other, we were fortunate to have companions close by who shared a fondness for almost all sports, especially baseball. As a devoted sibling, I lived by the universal little sister mantra established by older brothers, "get out of the way or learn to play." To borrow a phrase, I chose the latter and that made all the difference.

He pitched and I caught. He threw and I batted. He hit and I fielded. When we went to visit our like-minded city cousins, the four of us would go two on two. Gene and David lived near a real field, with bases and a fence and a dugout. To this day, we still recall quite vividly the time Scotty hit it over the fence and into a busy street. We all watched in absolute horror as a passing motorist stopped, opened his door, picked up the ball, and drove off. We threw our gloves to the ground in disgust and ran off to chase the car, though I'm still not sure why. All the way

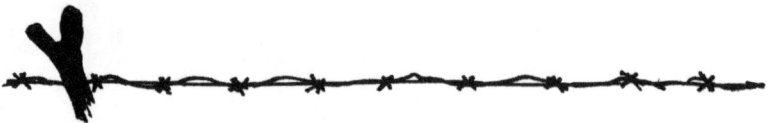

home, we mumbled about the drive-by looting. The incident was a definite reminder to me and to Scotty that living in a small town wasn't so bad after all. People did not steal baseballs where we lived.

Between us, Scotty and I had an entire set of the 1964 Yankees baseball trading cards: Mantle and Maris, Boyer and Richardson, Joe Pepitone and Tom Tresh, shortstop Tony Kubek, and catcher Elston Howard. On rainy days, we went to Scotty's room and built our own Yankee Stadium with our little brother and sister's building blocks, laid out the trading cards in the right positions, and played marble baseball. On summer weekends, we watched Yogi Bear cartoons on Saturday morning and watched Yogi Berra coach the Yankees on NBC's Saturday afternoon game of the week. Two Yogis in one day was pure entertainment.

Sandlot pick-up games were a mainstay after school and in the summer in our small town. The one concession that the guys made for me was the home run. If I hit it over the fence, it would count. The boys had to hit it not only over the fence but across the dirt road as well. My goal was to switch-hit home runs like Scotty, but I never could.

Despite the tomboy-ish life I led, I never doubted I was a girl and neither did the guys after the snake incident. It slithered onto the field and across my foot. My glove and my screams flew in the air as I ran home, not home plate, but H-O-M-E. Not until the chivalrous boys assured me their Louisville Sluggers had taken care of the creature did I return.

Throughout Little League, high school, and two years of college ball, Scotty remained my hero. I saw him struggle with his temper, with the "Establishment" of the 1970s that just knew long hair was a sign of worthless behavior, and with coaches who demeaned and rarely encouraged. These struggles, ironically, helped Scotty be the coach he became. Many grade school kids have grown to love baseball even more because of Scotty's approach to teaching a sport he has enjoyed for so long.

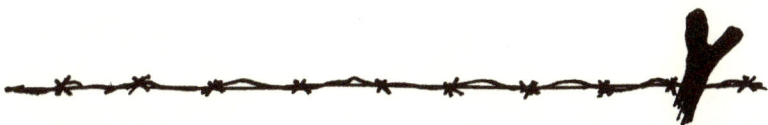

Baseball, October playoffs, and my brother just seem to go together. There are, of course, other threads that bind us such as a love for fudge and homemade ice cream. But this time of the year, it's always fun to know that someone is yelling at the television set as much as I am when the Yankees are in the playoffs. And gee whiz, if we could just find those trading cards, we could afford to buy out George Steinbrenner and have money left over to hire a private detective to track down that guy who stole our baseball.

—Sue Jane

 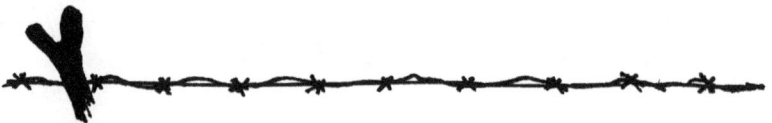

Capsule 68

Granny Rudd

Wth her daughter on one arm and her granddaughter on the other, Granny Rudd stepped down the aisle of the small church where her great grandson's wedding was being held. She preferred not to be handled, but the escort wasn't for balance; it was to make sure she did not wander off.

She was one of three great-grandparents at the wedding who suffered from Alzheimer's, and of the three, it was easy to tell which one had the ranching background. Skin weathered and wrinkled, legs bowed, and hands calloused, Granny Rudd's 93 years still reflected the spunk she had cultivated as a cowgirl many years ago. No disease was going to rob her of that.

But it had taken her from the ranch she had loved and the land where her grandfather and grandmother had come in the late 1800s. The irony was clear to me as I watched her fidget throughout the service and then turn antsy as the reception wore on.

Here she was, restricted but loved and cared for by a daughter and granddaughter who were giving her their best by sharing the long-term care. The very thing that Alzheimer's often brings on—the wandering spirit in and out of a faulty memory bank—is the very thing Granny Rudd had been allowed to do all of her life, to wander. On the ranch with her horse, her cattle, and her thoughts. Now, that wandering had to

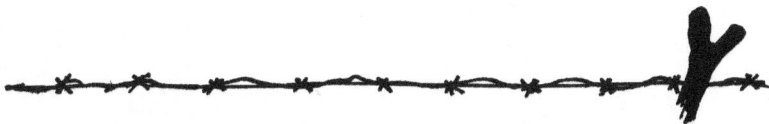

be prevented for her own safety. Alzheimer's is a cruel disease for anyone, but for those like Granny Rudd who have spent a lifetime roaming wide open spaces, the impact seems extra harsh.

When the wedding reception ended that Saturday night, she climbed in the back seat of the red pick-up truck, waiting for her granddaughter to drive her "home." Home to her ranch. Home to her big skies. Home where she could wander without someone grabbing her arm and pulling her back.

Granny Rudd has lived in heavenly realms for a long time; her streets of gold have been pastureland and windmills her ivory towers. She should feel right at home someday soon when the pearly gates open for her.

—Sue Jane

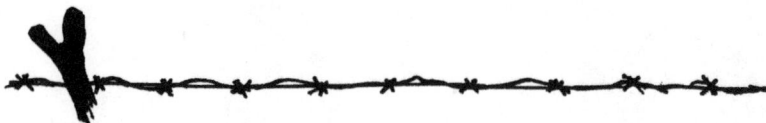

Capsule 69

A Vegetable Garden Recipe

You can spot one of two things in a rural family's backyard: either a vegetable garden or one of those inflatable swimming pools. When my daughters were younger, we had both. That definitely put us in the upper socio-economic class.

One summer, our garden was the biggest and the best in our area. Unusually good rains in June and early July helped keep us busy gathering, blanching, freezing, and then cooking those garden fresh vegetables.

As mentioned earlier, cooking wasn't my favorite activity. The girls' dad was the gardener; I was a reluctant participant who just went along to make peace. But I must admit there was one dish that I could really sink my teeth into. That's fried squash, okra, and potatoes all prepared in a cast iron skillet and served with warm cornbread.

Since I don't have a patent on garden vegetables, this recipe is public domain and now shared with our readers. Keep in mind that while you read this, my immediate family is laughing uncontrollably at the thought of my including recipes in this book.

1. Pick some okra and yellow crookneck squash from your garden. If you don't grow okra where you live, I'm sorry for you. You'll just have to buy some frozen. If you do not have

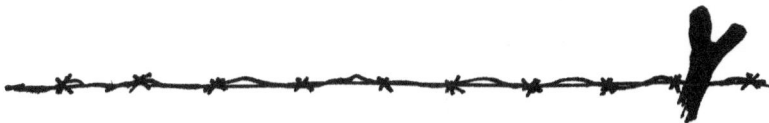

a garden, go get these ingredients out of your neighbor's. Country folks generally have that kind of agreement. If you aren't comfortable with that, then do the polite thing and ask. Strike a deal and say you'll cook for them if they will provide the vegetables.

2. Go buy three baking potatoes. If you have grown some in your garden, good for you.

3. While you are at the grocery store, get flour, cornmeal and canola oil. I know what you're thinking, "Why canola oil?" Just think of it as drinking a diet coke while you eat 10 slices of pizza.

4. Come home from the grocery store and take a good nap. This will make you feel rested before you slave over a hot stove. Preheat the oven while you take your power nap.

5. Wake up a few hours later.

6. Pour some canola oil in the cast iron skillet. Just how much depends on how many vegetables you are going to fry. Try a cup and a half.

7. Put the burner on low heat.

8. Start peeling the squash and then slice it in circle-like things. Soak them in a bowl of water.

9. Slice the ends off the okra with one of those cute paring knives.

10. Peel the potatoes. Then slice and dice them, too. Soak them in water.

Let's review: you have peeled squash, clipped okra, peeled and chopped up potatoes. Sounds like cruel and unusual punishment doesn't it?

11. Turn the heat up to medium on the oil.

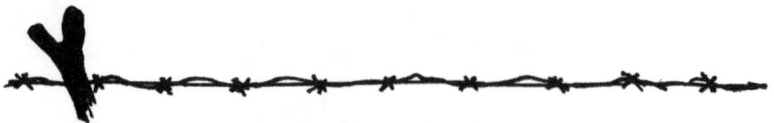

12. In a really big bowl, pour the squash and okra.
13. Pour in some cornmeal and flour mixture. Just guess on the amount—toss everything around until the squash and okra are covered with the mixture. If you need to add more cornmeal and flour, be my guest.
14. In a separate bowl (yes, you are going to use a lot of bowls for this recipe), pour your drained potatoes and add some flour. Toss this stuff around really well, and then add some salt and pepper.
15. Now mix the ingredients of the two bowls together.
16. Pour into cast iron skillet, cover, and fry.
17. Fry for 10-15 minutes on medium heat. You want the vegetables to be getting soft, and with the lid on, they will. Don't ask me why—it has something to do with physics.
18. Uncover and stir the vegetables. Put the lid back on.
19. Repeat #18 after 10-15 more minutes.
20. By now, the vegetables should be getting softer. Drain off some oil.
21. Turn up the heat. Leave lid on.
22. Check the vegetables in a couple of minutes and then use the metal spatula to turn them.
23. Drain off all oil.
24. Uncover and fry some more.
25. Turn as needed—meaning, don't let them burn.
26. When you finally get some of that great crusty brown stuff to show, you are almost finished. Drain one more time, turn down your heat, and cover again.

Hopefully, you already had your cast iron skillet cornbread baking in the oven—it should be ready by now. I hope you didn't cut corners and buy that deli cornbread or make cornbread sticks. The vegetable

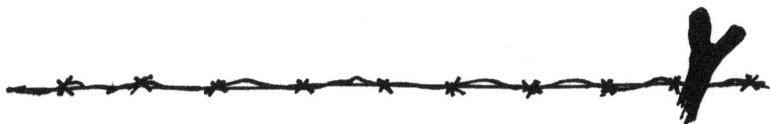

garden dish must be served with cornbread prepared in a cast iron skillet.

27. Add some more salt and pepper to the vegetables; cut the cornbread and add a lot of butter to each slice. I also like to add some mayonnaise on top of my cornbread—that's an old Arkansas trick my dad taught me.

28. Eat.

29. When you finish supper, soak those dishes in the dual-purpose inflatable pool.

There you have it, in 29 easy steps. A garden fresh vegetable recipe that explains what home cookin' is all about.

—Sue Jane

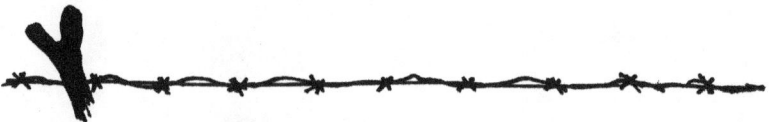

Capsule 70

There's Still a Lot of Love Here in These Troubled Fields

> If this rain can fall, these wounds can heal
> They'll never take our native soil
> But if we sell that new John Deere
> And then we'll work these crops with sweat and tears
> You'll be the mule, I'll be the plow
> Come harvest time we'll work it out
> There's still a lotta love, here in these troubled fields.

*S*inger/songwriter Nanci Griffith wrote this song in honor of an aunt and uncle who farmed for many years in the Texas Panhandle. It could have been written for any farming family. And it certainly has been true for my friends Ollie and Kent Holmes.

Their partnership has seen its share of troubled fields. The droughts, the ill-timed rains, and the hail and wind storms have damaged their cotton crop more often than they would like to remember. The loss of their 16-year-old son in 1986 almost damaged their spirits forever.

Not only has their love endured, the sweat and tears have irrigated growth in a relationship that began 40 years ago when two teenagers married and moved to the farm where they still live today in Borden County.

Their unique partnership was foreshadowed in the early 1960s when Kent reversed roles and walked Ollie off the football field where she had just finished playing in a powder puff football game. He drove

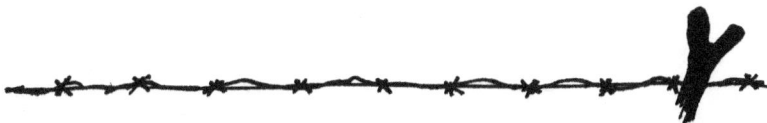

her home and then took her to the drive-in the next night, thus making official the courtship.

Their wedding took place on January 1, 1964. Everyone in Texas knows that January 1 is not just the start of new year. It is a football lover's buffet, and Ollie's family partook annually in the feast. The Kingston family were avid fans. If there was going to be a wedding to interrupt their day, it was going to take place at halftime. It did—halftime of the Texas-Alabama Cotton Bowl matchup in Dallas, Texas. Kent's family was wondering just what their son had done.

Today, Kent and Ollie are each other's biggest fans. Their partnership has not only sustained them but also nurtured so many others in the small county with a single school district.

The beneficiary list is long and the leadership roles are many that the two have filled in their lifelong commitment to each other and the county. Among them are the Junior Livestock Association, the school board, 4-H, the Baptist church and the Emergency Medical Service.

It is the latter that is the crown jewel, but it is the one community service that evolved from tragedy. That tragedy was the death of their teenage son. At the urging of friends who recognized both their need to deal with grief and the need for the emergency service in the county, Kent jumped into the emergency medical field. Ollie jumped on the tractor.

He would leave her in the field, waving at the tractor as he drove to classes from 30 minutes to an hour from their home. While Ollie was learning to farm, Kent was learning to splint, bandage, and transport people in the one ambulance the county had at that time.

This was just the beginning of something that Kent and Ollie readily admit came to "devour" them. Each turned to something that enabled them to grow instead of wither away in their sorrow.

Almost 20 years later, the Holmes continue to participate in the two activities that helped restore their troubled hearts after David's death.

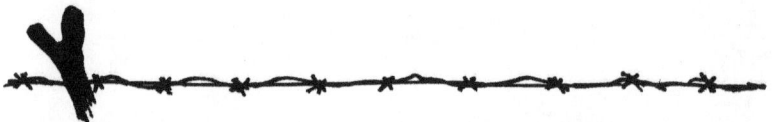

The best part is that they have become partners once again in the effort. Ollie still drives a tractor, but she also types Kent's tests for the many EMT and paramedic classes he volunteers to teach. Kent is back on a tractor, too, working alongside his wife in the cotton fields or pecan orchards.

The husband-wife team can be seen often in their fields just off Highway 180 twelve miles east of Gail. Or, they might be spotted on Friday nights at the football field where the local EMT volunteers are on call, wearing blue uniform shirts that Ollie has designed and made.

Together as a team, Kent and Ollie venture on. This year their cotton crop could be a bumper one. But, even if the weather doesn't cooperate, this farming family has proven that wounds can heal. A bumper crop of a lotta love is the key.

—Sue Jane

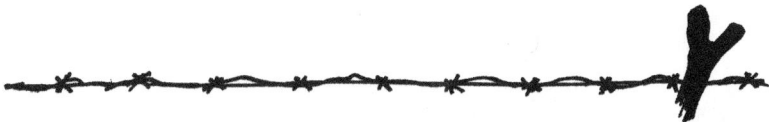

Capsule 71

Refrigerators, Sofas And Primary Care

*L*ooking at the ads in the Sunday paper, I realize that January is the time when consumers are urged to shop for big-ticket items such as refrigerators, freezers, and furniture. Intelligent consumers, we have standards; we seek value in these major purchases. I wonder why some of us are less discriminating when we shop for that other "big-ticket item"—primary health care.

Maybe part of the answer is that we don't think of seeking health care as a shopping activity. There are often fewer choices of health care providers nearby when we need them than there are brands of refrigerators or types of sofas. So, we wait until we are sick or worried and then just take what is available. That may mean that a person gets their health care mostly from emergency centers. Think about that—it's similar to waiting until your refrigerator gives out in July and then buying the only model on the showroom floor—at the July price. Worse yet, the available model doesn't have the same number of shelves as the one you had before. (That's the one that stopped completely on July 3.)

No self-respecting farmer or rancher wants to wait until they *have to* purchase the next tractor. No, we decide what we need and/or want and then carefully find the item that fills the bill. To me, primary health care is the same as the most basic type of equipment that a person uses. That is because primary care is the basic, everyday, type of health

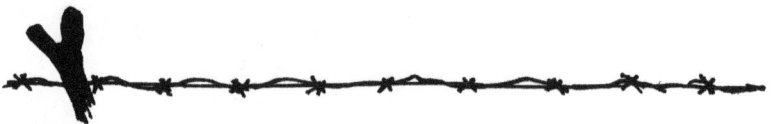

care that we all need. I am not talking about care provided in hospitals or by specialists. Primary care is just that, primary, first line. It is the refrigerator of health care. You would prefer not to be without one.

What choice do I have? you're thinking. There's only one clinic in town. My answer is this. If you are a good consumer of primary care services, you can have an influence on what is provided in that clinic. If the furniture store owner knows what the customer wants, they try to have it in stock, particularly if the owner knows the consumer *could* shop in the next town, thirty miles down the road. If you make your standards known and you do not get the primary care services (or sofa) that meets your expectations, you can shop around. That is the beauty of taking a "plan ahead" approach to primary health care, like planning ahead for other shopping.

Is that an idea worth thinking about? Let me help you get started. Here are some standards you could use in shopping for your primary care, in January rather than in July.

- The provider of primary care should be a person (or clinic) that you can think of as "home base." It should have services to treat minor and chronic illnesses *and* should emphasize health maintenance and health promotion. You should expect more than repairs. The primary care provider should help you avoid illness. You should receive education about routine maintenance you need such as immunizations, exams and screening. You should receive reminders about monitoring appropriate to your age and condition. You should get encouragement and education about healthy nutrition and habits.
- Your provider should keep a comprehensive record about you and your family. This information is essential to identify risks for illness and strengths to support health maintenance. For example, a good provider will ask who does the shopping and cooking

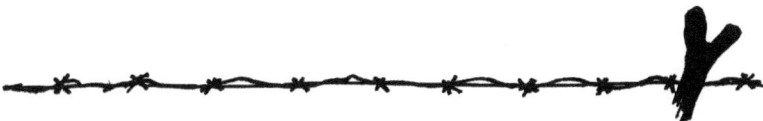

rather than just handing you a sheet of instructions for your diabetic diet.

◎ The history will include any care you receive from specialists to whom you are referred. Often, a patient will receive from several different specialists medications that could have dangerous interactions. If your provider is aware of you as a whole person, not just as a patient whose knee needs replacing, you are more likely to receive care that reflects that the quality of life is related to the whole person, not just the knee.

◎ Your provider should follow up. If you have lab work, you should get a letter or call about the results and their meaning. If you are ill, there should be a check on your improvement.

◎ The primary care provider should welcome you as a partner. Simply instructing a patient is insufficient. Questions must be encouraged and answers must be clear and complete.

That is a basic list of standards you can use as you choose your primary care. There will be other features you want that will be unique to you. Just as you look for a sofa with a particular fabric, you may prefer having a provider of a certain age or gender or other characteristics. Or, you may want a particular "brand." Nowadays, there are not only MDs (medical doctors) and DOs (doctors of osteopathy) who can be primary care providers, but also Physician Assistants and Nurse Practitioners. It's a little like Amana, Frigidaire or Kitchen Aid. The choice is yours. How you make these choices is important because your health is important. Primary health care should be chosen with the same degree of "savvy" that we apply to other big purchases. The quality of life can depend on it.

—Teddy

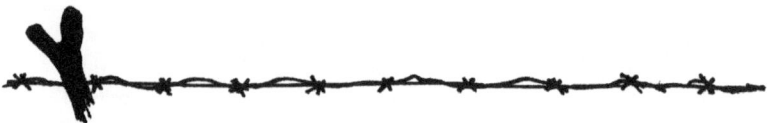

Capsule 72

Bet He's Gonna Be A Man Someday

Bob Wills probably didn't help matters when he sang "Roly Poly, daddy's little fatty, bet he's gonna be a man someday." The song described a child who ate everything in sight, was very active, and was Roly Poly. The notion was, "he's fat but that's fine because he will grow out of it." Could be that old Bob was reflecting an attitude that was fairly common when that tune was popular in the 1940s. Today we know that an overweight child has a strong chance of becoming an overweight adult. An analysis of national weight data completed in 2000, using information collected from 1988–1994, shows that 14 percent of children ages 6–11 and 12 percent of adolescents age 12–17 are overweight. Thirty-five percent of adults are overweight.

If the only problem caused by overweight were tight clothes, then we would not need to worry. But, research shows definite links between being overweight and high blood pressure, heart disease, and the development of type two diabetes.

Remember when the tables of ideal weights had three categories—small, medium, and large frame? That probably encouraged some folks to fall back on "I have large bones" as the reason for their weight. And it is true that some of us are genetically destined to have a larger skeleton than others. Scientists have developed a better way to identify a range of desirable weight for a person. The Body Mass Index is

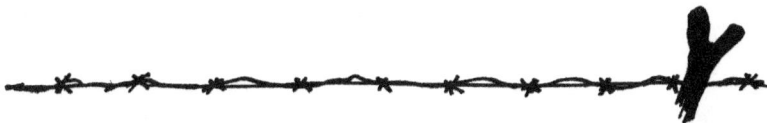

calculated by a formula that takes both height and weight into account. Desirable weight for an adult is within a range of the BMI numbers, not a narrow five-pound range for "body frame." The range of desirable BMI is between 18.5 and 24.9 for adults. This takes into account differences in both skeleton and muscular development and is suitable for use across the adult age span.

The same approach is used for children starting at age two. But, there is an added step. In order to account for the fact that children are growing, after the index number is determined based on height and weight, it is plotted on a chart for age. Norms developed across large numbers of children are printed as a series of lines to show the percentiles from 5th to 97th. A child whose BMI number plots above the 95th percentile for age is overweight, no matter how cute those pudgy arms and legs are. Above the 85th percentile is a risk of overweight. By that standard, Roly Poly would be considered overweight only if he had a Body Mass Index higher than 95 of 100 kids his age. Maybe he just has chubby cheeks!

Suppose that he is overweight. What can a parent or grandparent do to lessen R.P.'s chances of becoming an overweight, hypertensive diabetic someday? Here are a few ideas:

1. Increase physical activity. Limit video games and television. Encourage walking, running, and cycling as methods of transportation, preferably encouraging by example.
2. Reduce caloric intake. A growing child needs nutrients, so the only desirable way to reduce calories is to reduce non-nutritive calories. Those are in the foods up on the top of the Food Pyramid, found most often in sweets and fats. There's no reason to abandon pizza entirely or to completely withhold all potato chips. But, make those things an occasional treat rather than an every day item. Replace soft

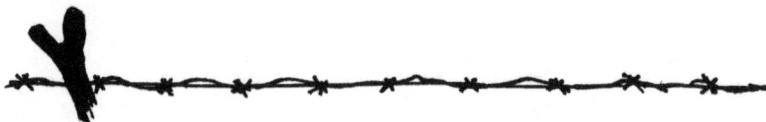

drinks with water. If a soft drink is chosen, how about something smaller than the 32 ounce HUGE that is sold as a bargain? Food has many meanings beyond nourishment. Social activities revolve around food; food is often used as reward; from infancy food equals comfort. So, changing food intake for a child is best accomplished by changing food-related behavior for the whole family. The potential Roly Poly does not think that he or she is being deprived or punished by being fed differently if the whole family observes healthy eating patterns.

3.   When the child is seen by a health care provider, make certain that the Body Mass Index for Age chart is used to plot their growth each year. Ask about the results. Better yet, check for yourself. If you have Internet access, you can print the BMI tables and the chart to plot BMI for Age from the website at www.cdc.gov/nccdphp/dnpa/bmi/bmi-for-age.htm. There you can learn more about weight, healthy eating and recommended physical activity.

The little guy that inspired Bob Wills' song was probably adorable. But he would probably be healthier today if instead of "eat an apple pie as quick as you can wink an eye," someone had taught him to just eat the apple.

—Teddy

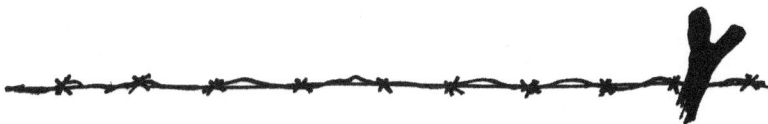

Capsule 73

Swallows Don't Worry About Bar Ditches

I don't know much about swallows except that at least one pair builds a mud-based nest on our front porch every summer. This summer they are the parents of two. The babies' fuzzy heads are just visible over the edge of the nest. It won't be long before those youngsters join their parents in aiming at the chairs where we sit to enjoy the sunset.

Watching them today, I wasn't thinking much about strategic chair placement. (They are very accurate hitting any target with their droppings.) Rather, I was thinking about what a Nurse Practitioner friend had told me recently of two cases she had in Emergency. Two teens (under driving age) had rolled the family car on a county road. While both of those youngsters had survived, the crash resulted in some serious injuries. "What were they doing driving?" she asked. My offhand response was, "We're in the country. They drive as soon as they can see over the steering wheel."

The swallows have a job raising their two. There's feeding, protecting, and teaching them to fly. They put a lot of effort into those concerns. Fortunately for them, they don't have to deal with teaching them to drive, setting rules about when they can drive, or worrying while they are out driving. My response to my colleague, offhand as it was, reflected both tradition and an unresolved health problem for those in rural areas. The tradition is based on necessity. Kids do begin to drive

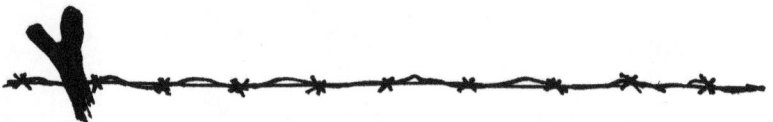

when very young, often to help get the numerous chores completed. First it's just, "Steer the pickup through and I'll shut the gate." Then they want their own pickup. So many tasks on the farm or ranch require driving some sort of vehicle that driving becomes an essential skill. It is natural to encourage any aptitude or interest in driving.

As for the health problem, your family has been fortunate if it has had no major accidents due to underage drivers. National data, from the Centers for Disease Control's Center for Injury Prevention state that in 2001 (most recent report), more than 4,700 teens ages 16–19 died from motor vehicle accidents. For all causes of death of teenagers, two out of five were attributed to motor vehicle accidents, more than any other cause of death. Though the death numbers are distressing, the overall injury and damage figures are far higher. The cost attributed to vehicle accidents with drivers ages 15–20 in 2002 was $48 billion.

The Injury Prevention Center suggests that primary reasons for these vehicle related injuries and deaths are: inexperience, low rates of safety belt use, alcohol use, and nighttime driving. They cite evidence to support these as sources of the problem.

I do not doubt them, but those factors do not take into account other conditions peculiar to rural areas. County roads and turn-rows are frequented by tractors and other large vehicles moving implements. The visibility for both the "ag-driver" and the passenger vehicles in the vicinity is impaired and reduced speed is necessary. Tell "reduced speed" to a teen driver and see how that is interpreted. Those county roads are usually dirt, gravel or caliche-surfaced. Traversing them in wet weather demands good decision-making skills even for experienced drivers. The inexperienced tend to over-correct, so that one wheel entering a pothole or a muddy slide becomes the source of a complete rollover.

The curves on those roads are seldom as well banked as on the Farm-to-Markets or the State Highways. I recall a late night game that was a common diversion in my hometown when I was a teen. It involved

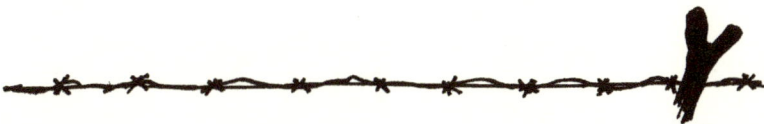

turning off the headlights and negotiating the dirt roads at high speeds. The risk (and the excitement) was heightened by the flat curves and the presence of deep bar ditches on either side of the road. And I wasn't even the driver!

One of the remedies for the health hazards of teenage driving suggested by the CDC is for laws requiring a graduated approach to licensing drivers. A period of driving with supervision precedes solo driving. Limits are placed on driving at night. That may help in some places, but since young drivers in rural areas often are not licensed anyway, the remedy with a greater chance of success is for parents to make and enforce rules. Don't let them drive off your property until they are properly licensed. Require the seatbelt. Disapprove actively of driving under the influence of alcohol.

Swallows let the young fly when they are developmentally ready. Until then, they guard them carefully. Those nestlings demand food, but never ask for the pickup keys, "just to go get a Coke." Swallow parents have it made. There's only the eight foot drop from the nest to worry about, not miles of dirt road and deep bar ditches.

—Teddy

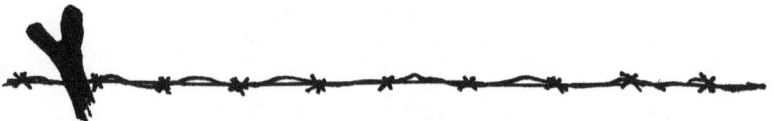

Capsule 74

Every Occupation Has Its Hazards

A gray-brown pall hangs low over the pens, forming and rising as the cattle pace the perimeter of the enclosures. Destination indefinite, they travel the limits from the feed bunks to their bovine neighbors' fences and back, their afternoon journey. It's a common sight at feedlots any time the wind lays, this cloud of particles so thick and murky. The pen rider coughs, sneezes, and mutters an expletive describing the odor. It's an occupational hazard.

Two teenaged boys, equipped with grain scoops and rubber boots, have a job today. They are cleaning out chicken coops, removing manure, feathers, and other accumulated poultry debris. They took the job because the wage was more than the minimum. As they wade in and scoop, trading ideas about weekend plans, one tells the other his chest feels tight. His friend's response is, "Yeah, well, my eyes are watering non-stop. How'd you like to be a chicken and live in here? Now get up and scoop. We can be finished in another hour." Not sympathetic.

Similar scenes—respiratory reactions upon exposure to animal hair, feather, feces, urine, hay, grain, silage and dust—occur daily where farmers and ranchers do their work. Occupational hazards abound.

The sneezing, coughing, and nose blowing are mainly annoyances for some people. All that mucous production signals that

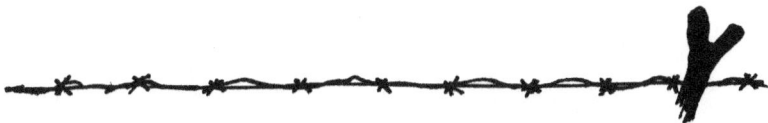

the protective mechanisms in the respiratory passages are working, rejecting irritants. But, the hazards created by these situations can be more serious. There are illnesses that can result and for some, the damage can be long lasting. Farmer's Lung disease and Organic Dust Toxic Syndrome are worth knowing about when you work in agriculture. In both of these illnesses, the culprits are dust and molds.

Farmer's Lung is a type of inflammation of the lung caused initially by an allergic hypersensitivity to molds commonly found in stored grain or silage. While only some people are "genetically engineered" to have the allergic reaction, those who are will usually have symptoms with each exposure to the offending particles. The symptoms may be mistaken for a cold or flu. They include chills, low-grade fever, fatigue, cough, chest congestion, and a feeling of shortness of breath or constriction. The illness can last from one to seven days, unless it is complicated by a bacterial infection in the lungs that can become pneumonia. One problem is that the person may not make the connection between the inhalant exposure and the subsequent illness. Thinking it is a cold or flu, they may have increasingly severe reactions to subsequent exposures because they are unaware of the need to protect themselves due to their allergic sensitivity. Repeated reactions can eventually cause lasting lung damage.

Organic Dust Toxic Syndrome can happen to anyone (allergic or not) who inhales a large amount of dust and molds at any one exposure. Those boys at the chicken coop are candidates. Even if this one experience convinces them they want a career in accounting (also not without occupational hazards), the day-long dose of the "fowl" dust can be enough to cause illness.

The symptoms are similar to Farmer's Lung and the course of one to seven days of illness is similar, as well. If you do develop an illness within one to seven days after exposure to agricultural molds and dust, and you do not improve rapidly, see your health care provider. Report that the illness follows the dust/mold exposure. That information

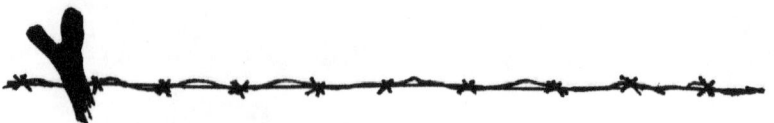

is important in assuring the correct treatment. Leaving agriculture is not the only answer to dealing with these illnesses. Preventive steps are the most important:

- Keep the dust and mold from being liberated into the air by wetting any area that is to be cleaned or moved.
- Areas where dust and mold form, such as livestock enclosures or grain and silage storage, should be cleaned frequently to reduce the accumulation of the mold and dust.
- Wear a respirator with sufficient filtering ability to block out the particles. A single-thickness paper mask that will work when you're mowing grass is not enough.

Every occupation has its hazards. Whether the occupation is farming, ranching, or accounting, those hazards can spell trouble if we are not aware and if we do not take preventive action.

—Teddy

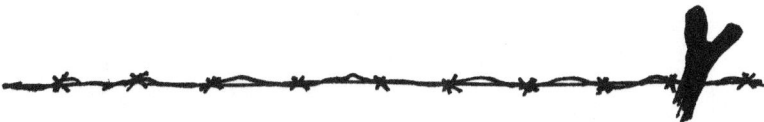

Capsule 75

Taking Stock

*E*gads! I thought. Since no one I know actually *says* Egads, I didn't, but the sight before me was enough to prompt an outburst. Asked to get a small bandage for my friend to apply to a cut on her daughter's finger, I opened their bathroom medicine cabinet. I was shocked as only a nurse can be to see that this family was suffering—from an acute need to Take Stock.

In this case, the contents of the cabinet needed careful review. Taking stock could mean considering what was there that should not be and what might be missing. There was nothing missing. No room for the kitchen sink, but I was surprised to see it absent. I overcame my urge to begin tossing pill bottles. I said not a word when I delivered the bandage. But, rest assured, I will mention this to my friend very soon. While the memory of that cabinet is fresh, let me offer some pointers on taking stock—in the home medicine cabinet.

Although thriftiness is admirable, some things should not be saved. The top item on the "throw away" list is any partially used prescription medicine that is not currently prescribed. The major culprit here is leftover antibiotics. There are two reasons. First, specific antibiotics are used for specific illness because the bacteria that cause one illness often differ from those causing another. So, saving the medicine "in case I need an antibiotic" is not good reasoning. Second, there should not be

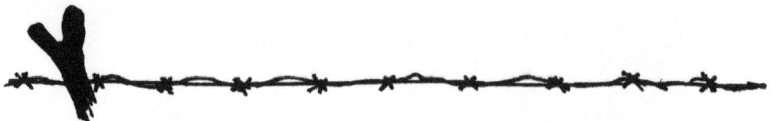

any leftover antibiotics. When you have a prescription for an antibiotic, the whole prescription should be taken. Research suggests that at least part of the reason for the development of antibiotic-resistant bacteria is partial treatment that does not effectively "finish off" the pathogen.

Another reason for the development of these super germs is the overuse of antibiotics. The best course of action is to only take antibiotics when an illness is bacterial (not viral-antibiotics do not kill viruses) and when your health care provider says they are actually needed. And when you start the antibiotic, finish it. Whew, glad I got that off my chest!

Besides antibiotics, any other prescription that is not currently in use should be discarded if it was purchased more than one year ago unless there is an indication it has not passed its expiration date. Potency can be affected.

The other prescription item that should be destroyed rather than stored is pain medication. Not only can outdated medication lose its effectiveness, but its presence also can be a temptation to children who enjoy experimenting.

Non-prescription items should be reviewed also. Research from Yale University School of Medicine resulted in a warning about certain over-the-counter drugs. The Food and Drug Administration determined that phenylpropanolamine is unsafe for continued use due to risk of hemorrhagic strokes. This drug is in diet pills and some cold and cough preparations. Read the labels. If you see PPA or phenylpropanolamine in your favorite cough syrup, dispose of it immediately. A similar warning was issued on ephedra, often labeled as ma huang. This is in body building supplements and in some "natural" diet preparations.

Now that some space is clear in that cabinet, look for laxatives. Why are they there? Better to correct bowel irregularity with increased fluid, fruits, and fiber. If the problem persists, a fiber supplement containing cellulose or psyllium would be far gentler and less likely to cause dependence. If those remedies don't work, you should see a health

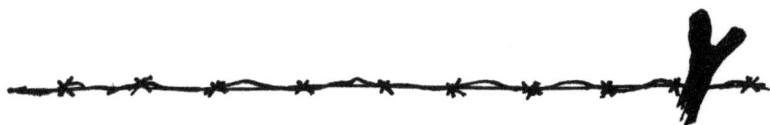

care provider rather than drink milk of magnesia as a nightly toddy.

What is that up on the top shelf? If it's a mercury thermometer, plan to discard it, also. A broken thermometer will spill mercury, a health hazard. Even though you have no *plans* to break the thermometer, it is safer, particularly if children are in the household, to have a battery-operated thermometer. When you get rid of a mercury thermometer, do not put it in the trash. As you probably know the danger from mercury is most potent when vapor from it is inhaled or from skin contact. Take it to a health care facility and ask that it be disposed of as labeled hazardous waste.

There are lots of other things that are stored in medicine cabinets that are none of my business. I would never urge anyone to toss out a lipstick in a favorite color, even if it is five years old. And it is surely beyond my scope and space here to suggest every item that should be there. But, there is one last item I do want to mention. If there are children in the house, consider how fascinating the medicine chest might be to them. Remember how they climb. With kids around, taking stock should also include considering the best childproof location for all medicines.

—Teddy

 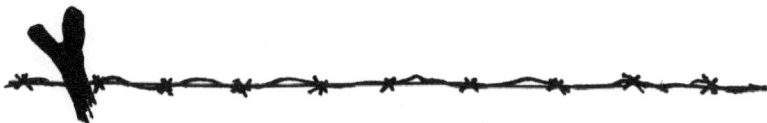

Capsule 76

Some Things Are Clearer Than Others

*M*edications and age—that's what set me thinking about what is clear and what is not so clear. Since many of us take prescription medications and/or vitamins or herbal supplements, those things that are not so clear are important to know about.

First, it is clear when a child is younger than about twelve, special care is needed when giving drugs. Children weigh less than adults; the major organs affecting the metabolism and excretion of medicines (liver and kidneys) are not fully mature; and body composition, particularly ratio of fat to lean muscle mass, is different than in adults. Those factors all affect decisions about dose and type of medication. There are abilities that children develop only as they grow older which also affect those decisions. Such abilities include swallowing pills or capsules; reading, comprehending, and following instructions; and recognizing and reporting side effects. All of these considerations have an impact on the choice of medicines and the ways they are given. It is also clear that adjustments such as smaller doses, liquids instead of pills, and administration of the drugs by an adult are all necessary for children.

Not so clear is the point at which consideration of changes at the other end of the age spectrum should begin. When, exactly, does one merit the description "elderly"? Does that arrive along with the first Social Security check? Or does "elderly" fit only when a person becomes frail?

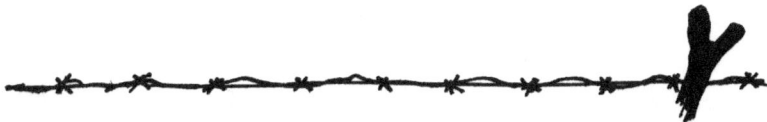

The issues related to medications and the elderly are important, just as important as for children. And, just as with children, many of the concerns are related to physiologic differences. The age at which these precautions must be observed vary with the individual. Some are experiencing the physical changes by 65. Others change more slowly. Eventually, we all will change.

One major change is in the ratio of lean muscle mass and body water to body fat. The elderly body has less water and muscle and more fat. As a result, drugs that are soluble in fat deposit for longer periods of time and have longer effects. Examples are such drugs as tranquilizers and sedative-hypnotics such as "sleeping pills." The dose of one of these that was effective and safe for a 35 year-old may create confusion and cause a fall and fractured hip for an elderly person.

Reduced body water composition also changes the effect of water-soluble drugs, such as alcohol. As a result of the reduced volume of water, the alcohol (or other water-soluble drug) is increased in the blood stream and is therefore more potent than the same amount (dose) would be in a younger adult.

The efficiency of the kidneys and liver change with age. As circulation slows or chronic disease affects these organs, their ability to metabolize and excrete medicines is reduced. As a result, smaller, less frequent doses of medications are needed for the elderly.

Over time, on the way to becoming elderly, a person is likely to have been prescribed medicines that are continuous, for chronic conditions such as arthritis, diabetes, or high blood pressure. As each drug is added, the potential for side effects increases as does the possibility of dangerous interactions among the drugs. This hazard is increased by the common practice of seeing several different health care providers and having no one provider who is aware of all the medications that a person is receiving. Using one pharmacy for all prescriptions can reduce the danger associated with having multiple prescribers, if the pharmacist

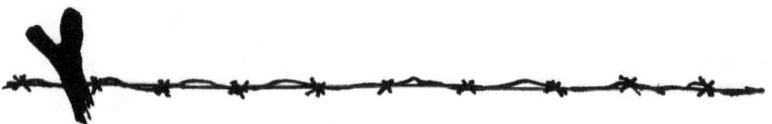

is careful to keep a profile of medications each person is taking. But, all too often, the patient is treated with drug samples or uses several different pharmacies so no comprehensive list is maintained. One other thing that seems clear to me is that all of us who are in the middle, no longer children and not yet elderly, can take some steps to be sure that there are fewer problems related to medicines and age. We can:

- ✪ Ask a lot of questions about any medication prescribed for any member of the family, whatever the age. Read the drug handouts provided by the pharmacist. Ask the health care provider why a prescription is recommended and what alternatives there are.
- ✪ Review our own and family members' medications at least every 6 months and when any new item is added, be certain that what is being taken is needed and that correct dose and schedule are being used. Include in this review all over-the-counter preparations and vitamins and herbals.

—Teddy

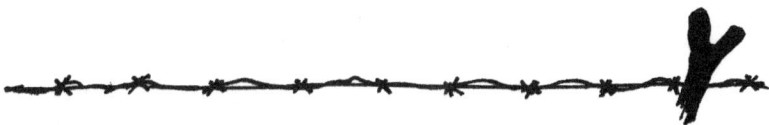

Capsule 77

Don't Let Them Avoid Getting These Facts

*D*o you know one of those men who puts off seeing a health care provider unless he feels really sick? Does the idea of a regular checkup seem to be stored near the track in his brain that says, "If it ain't broke..."? Does that seem a little inconsistent with the meticulous attention to preventive maintenance he lavishes on farm and ranch machinery?

Well, it's understandable. If there are no knocks and pings, it's easy to put off making an appointment. And then there's the fact that some parts of the "fact gathering" he's subjected to during a good checkup are a little less than pleasant. Actually, there's only one part of the exam that tends to be considered universally unpleasant. It's the digital rectal exam (DRE). In the words of one man I recently saw in clinic, "As soon as I saw the doctor put on her glove, my blood pressure went up. I told her I didn't have high blood pressure and didn't need any medicine for that, but I sure did need her to put that glove away."

Unpleasant? Yes, a little. Important? Very. Here's the reason. The DRE, in conjunction with the PSA (prostate specific antigen, a blood test) provides facts necessary to determine whether further testing for prostate cancer is needed.

Prostate cancer is the second most common cancer in men in the U.S., exceeded only by skin cancer. As a cause of cancer-related death

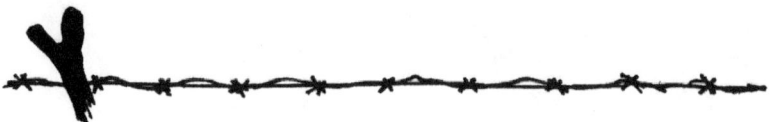

in men, prostate cancer is second only to lung cancer. The American Cancer Society estimates that near 189,000 new cases of prostate cancer would be diagnosed each year and approximately 30,000 men will die of the disease each year. But, with early detection and treatment, prostate cancer doesn't have to be deadly. Fewer than 10% of men with prostate cancer who are treated die within five years of the diagnosis.

Age and race make a difference in incidence of prostate cancer. African Americans have the highest rates, followed by whites, Hispanics, American Indians, and Asian/Pacific Islanders, in that order. Incidence is higher in men over 65, with about 80% of diagnosed prostate cancer in men over 65. Those are the facts about American men as a group.

A man's *own* facts are the ones that matter most to him. To get those facts, he needs the exam and the blood test, *both*. Men with first-degree relatives who have had prostate cancer or who are African American should begin "collecting the facts" around age 40. Other should get this information annually beginning at age 50.

The PSA:

The PSA tests for the amount of a chemical normally produced by glandular prostate cells. If these cells are damaged by infection or trauma or altered by cancer, the substance can leak into the bloodstream. Because the substance is produced normally and can be affected by conditions other than cancer, it is not cancer-specific. It is only one fact. The normal value, overall, for PSA is less than 4 nanograms/milliliter with 4–10 considered borderline. But, since PSA varies normally with age, reference values by age are as follows:

Age	PSA
40-49	less than 1.5
50-59	less than 2.5
60-69	less than 4.5
70-79	less than 7.5

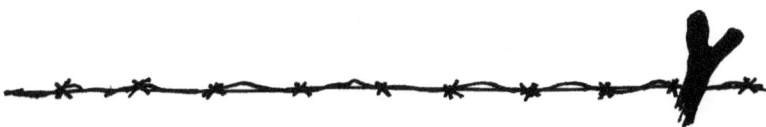

The clinician can interpret the results, based on age and on the normal range of values for the laboratory that performs the test.

The DRE:

The DRE is a direct examination by the clinician, using the index finger to feel through the front of the rectum the texture and size of the back portion of the prostate. If the prostate is hard, not smooth, or is enlarged, these are abnormal findings.

If either fact (DRE or PSA) is not normal that's a signal that further tests should be performed—not necessarily that cancer is present. Additional tests are usually performed upon referral to a urologist and may include blood tests for infection, repeat PSA with a determination of percent of "free PSA," ultrasound, and/or needle biopsy.

Here's the good new. Statistics show that if the U.S. male population over age 50 were all tested with PSA, 85% would have normal results. Of the other 15% who have an abnormal PSA and would need further testing, twelve would not have prostate cancer. And for those men who did have cancer, early detection would increase the likelihood of a positive treatment result. That early detection is one more reason for the preventive maintenance approach, a good reason to have regular checkups. If a man in your family should have a prostate exam, tell him, "Don't let the sight of a rubber glove make you avoid getting the facts."

—Teddy

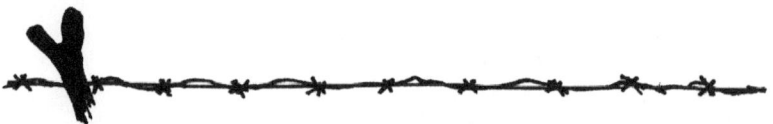

Capsule 78

My Othermama Knew Best

"You're gonna catch epizootic!" I'm remembering the warning I heard so often in my early years. Othermama (my maternal grandmother) used the threat of "epizootic" as the consequence I would reap from any number of not-too-clean practices in which I might engage. Playing with cats, not washing my hands before eating, picking at scabs—and probably picking my nose—all were reasons for her to raise the possibility of that direst of all diseases, "epizootic." But she never once said I shouldn't drink the water at her house. That water was supplied by a cistern that collected run-off from the roof. From the cistern, it was transported by hand pump to a bucket with a red-rimmed enameled dipper we *all* drank from.

I know now that "epizootic" is not the name of a specific disease. And I know, also, that I am probably fortunate never to have caught something from drinking that water.

Remembering that dipper and the water at her house, where indoor plumbing didn't arrive until 1955, started me thinking about the water sources that many of us use in rural areas. Are we in danger of "catching epizootic" or of suffering some ill effects from our water? The answer is yes. For the 15% of rural residents whose water supply is a private well, spring, or cistern, two preventive approaches are important. First, understand your water system, its sources, and potential

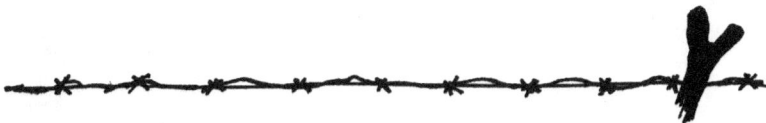

contaminants. Second, have your water tested regularly, at least annually.

Since the Joneses are in that 15%, I have done a bit of searching for information to help with those approaches. Perhaps the facts will be useful to you or someone you know, as well.

Both well and spring water come directly from underground sources. Any underground source is fed by above ground water that seeps in across a leach field in the watershed area for that particular source. Since I don't know much about geology, I won't try to explain this any more than to say that as the water seeps underground, fed by rain and run-off from higher ground, it can acquire both natural and human-caused sources of contamination. Whatever is happening to that water as it passes across the ground miles away can affect the well on your property. As the water courses downward, some of the contaminants may be left behind in the layers of earth it passes through. But, there's no guarantee that this natural filtration will eliminate all contaminants. In fact, in some areas, the earth itself may be a source of natural compounds dangerous to humans if they are in high concentrations. Those include boron, arsenic, magnesium, calcium, chloride, selenium, and radon.

But, the likelihood of natural contamination is far less than that of human-caused sources. Fertilizer, pesticides, herbicides, and insecticides applied to fields or drained into storm drains or directly on the ground can travel into underground water. Leaking underground chemical storage tanks or chemical spills at industrial sites can also add unhealthy chemical compounds to the water traveling downward to the underground sources we tap. Sources of bacterial and viral contamination are human and animal manure from poorly constructed or poorly drained septic systems and from concentrated animal production operations. While there are protective state and federal rules and regulations for activities involving each of these hazards, sometimes they are not followed or are not fully effective.

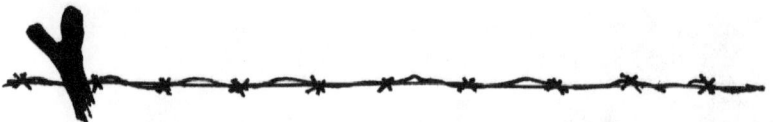

Since cisterns are reservoirs for rainwater, the main trouble sources with them occur in storage or in transport from storage to human use (the communal dipper, for example). The same hazards apply to well and spring water after it is captured for use. Old pipes can have holes that permit contaminants to enter. Or they may be welded with lead, a dangerous contaminant. Holding tanks or cisterns that are not properly sealed can admit rodents. Filters may be missing or may not be changed often enough.

Having said all that, it is evident why regular testing is important. Contact your State Health Department for information on labs that provide the testing. For additional information on the quality of private water sources, a useful website is www.uwex.edu/farmasyst. From there you can link to information provided through programs in your home state.

Illnesses from contaminated water are often gastrointestinal. But neurological and other serious problems are caused by some of the contaminants as well. Any of us can be affected, but children, the elderly and those with compromised immune systems such as transplant patients are most vulnerable. Take preventive action. No one needs to "catch epizootic."

—Teddy

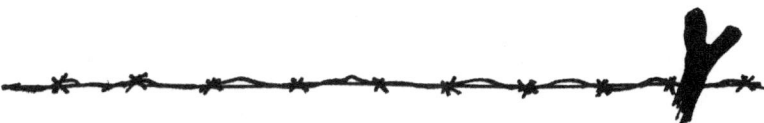

Capsule 79

Another Form Of Stress Reduction

Stories travel, gaining momentum as they roll along. A tumbleweed reminds me as it collects a bit of unharvested cotton lint. Rolling along in the West Texas wind, it gathers a plastic bag, a devil's claw, a piece of dried manure. Lodging on a fence, it's more than when it began its trek. It's the same with stories, particularly those of medical encounters. So, when I heard recently about an acquaintance spending three hours in an emergency department providing information before receiving treatment, I attributed a couple of those hours to the effect of repeated retelling, rolling along. But, I thought, regardless of time elapsed on the clock on the treatment room wall, any time delaying treatment seems interminable, especially when pain and fear are involved. Serious stress there.

Can that be prevented? I wondered. After thinking about the information that a health care provider needs in order to give competent care, I think the answer is—yes, it's partly preventable.

As with any preventive action, this will take a little effort in advance of the problem. Maybe you'd do what I'm about to suggest instead of the usual New Year's diet resolution. That would be a refreshing change, wouldn't it?

Here's the idea. Compile a brief vital information and health history record for each family member. I'll help by outlining the categories

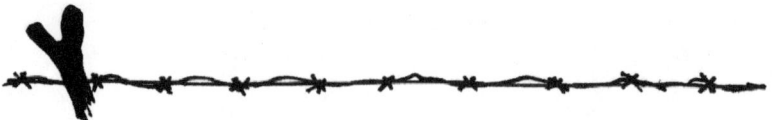

and explaining the content for each one. You'll compile the information, make two copies and put one in a file at home and one in the billfold or purse of each adult. Flip a coin to decide who carries the kids' papers. Update at least once each year.

You may wonder why you need to do this if you usually see the same health care provider. "He or she has my records. Why do I need to carry another piece of paper?" The answer? Emergencies don't always send you to your regular provider or to a familiar hospital. And even the person who's treated you for years can speed your care in an emergency if they don't have to read backward through thirty years of records to extract history.

There's nothing revolutionary about what I'm suggesting. There are a few health care systems that now provide their members the convenience of having this type of information stored on a computer-readable card. Those of us who don't have the digital version can still have our own, complete, and up-to-date information in our pockets. All it takes is a bit of time and effort invested in stress reduction.

If the idea of compiling the information seems like a large task, consider this. Compile each family member's material as a birthday present. That would spread the work throughout the next year. Many young adults (your children?) have relied on parents to be their historians. They put infectious childhood illnesses and broken bones out of their minds in favor of present-moment concerns. Suddenly one day, they are adults and should have that information for themselves. Can you think of a more useful gift? For an older family member, having the information handy can save hours and errors of omission in an emergency or a visit to a specialist.

If I've convinced you that developing portable health history is worthwhile, we'll begin. We'll start with category headings. Later we'll complete the content of the sections.

You'll use the same format for each person, so make copies of

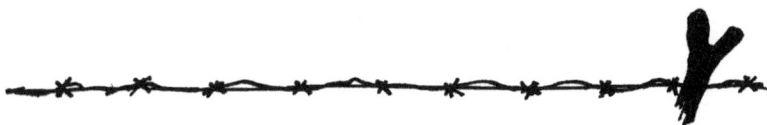

the category headings and fill in the blanks as you collect information. You can save carrying space by copying on "reduce" to the smallest size that the "owner" can read.

Categories:
Personal Data
Family/Social data
Current Health Status
Immunizations
Childhood Illnesses
Surgical History including fractures
Medical/Mental Health Conditions

A warning is in order. Even though you present this information when you go for emergency or specialist care, the competent provider will still ask questions, not only about the current illness, but also to confirm the history your record contains. You will have the advantage of an organized complete set of facts. That will save time and frustration. And that reduces stress.

—Teddy

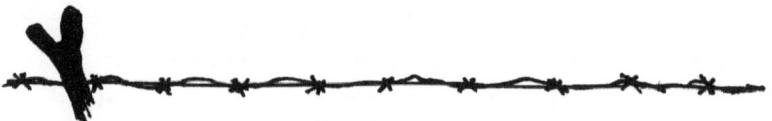

Capsule 80

The Rest Of The Story

*E*arlier I urged you to compile a portable personal health history. The final note suggested the key categories. This installment specifies essential content for each category.

Personal Data: Full name, date of birth, height, usual weight, eye and hair color, social security number, emergency notification name and number, marital status, insurance coverage including policy numbers, religious affiliation, current occupation, military service, recent foreign travel, and name and number of usual primary health care provider.

Current Health Status: This section can be important for providers in that it offers a view of usual function which can be compared to the current condition. Include the following:

Known allergies

Assistive devices (dentures, eyeglasses or contacts, cane, hearing aid, walker, etc.)

Current medications: (include name of drug and doses, also vitamin or herbal supplements and medications taken only as needed such as over the counter pain medication, antihistamines, or antacids and frequency of use)

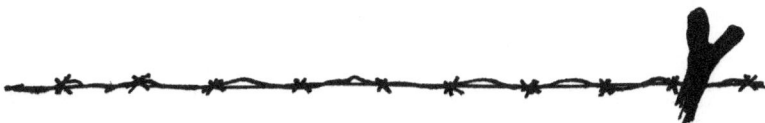

Patterns describing a usual day or week: Usual amount of daily sleep and rest, meal pattern, special diet, exercise, pattern of bowel and bladder elimination, and other habits such as caffeine, nicotine and alcohol use. For example, 1 package of chewing tobacco/ week for 50 years. Including this latter information can be important since sudden deprivation of nicotine, caffeine, or alcohol can create symptoms such as headaches or nervousness which may be wrongly attributed to other causes if the provider is unaware.

Immunizations: Include dates of last immunizations for adults for tetanus, pertussis, smallpox, hepatitis B, influenza and pneumonia. For a child until age 12, it's useful to keep handy the immunization records that will indicate the currency and completeness of all the currently recommended childhood immunizations. If you've recently served in the military or traveled abroad, you should have a record of the related immunizations. Any tuberculosis test date in the past two years and results should also be noted.

Childhood Illnesses: For some, childhood is so far past it's a dim memory. But some childhood infectious illnesses can result in later health problems. Examples are glomerulonephritis (kidney) or rheumatic heart disease can result from frequent strep throat. List all childhood infectious diseases the subject had including measles, mumps, three day measles, whooping cough, diphtheria, chickenpox, polio and any frequent childhood illnesses such as strep throat, middle ear infections, or asthma.

Surgical History Including Fractures: The simplest method here is to make a table as below:

Date	Surgery or other	Reason	Outcome
1954	gallbladder	stones	o.k.

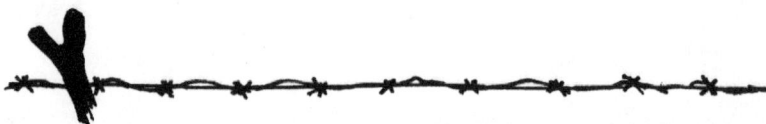

| 1961 | broken rt. Femur | horse fall | pin in |

If female, include pregnancies and whether a live birth resulted. Don't worry about using correct medical terms, the provider can interpret if you have the history in place.

Other Medical or Mental Health Treatment: This section is for illnesses/treatments in the *past*. Use a table as in the example below.

First date of problem	Illness	Treatment	Outcome
1971	pneumonia	antibiotic	resolved
1994	depression	medication	continue med

Mention also if you ever received a blood transfusion as part of medical or surgical treatment.

Current Health Problems: The final segment is for health problems currently under treatment. Since you've listed medication in a prior section, this is a brief list of current problems *being treated*. Examples might be diabetes, high blood pressure, hyperlipidemia, or asthma.

That's it! You might notice that the process of recalling the information causes some discomfort as it you put it in print. Were you uneasy about writing that you get no regular exercise, that you use antacids every day, or your weight? Maybe that's because these are areas where you need to improve. Trust your discomfort to guide you to new goals. And meanwhile, you have a summary of health information that can be a boon to any health care provider you see. He or she can be far more effective in dealing with new problems efficiently if you have this information as a beginning point for the detective work necessary for competent diagnosis and treatment.

—Teddy

Capsule 81

A Spa Is Where You Find It

I knew a woman once who had really arrived. She had worked her way, quite literally, through the ranks of the nursing departments at a couple of hospitals; staff nurse, nurse manager, staff educator. When the opportunity to enter hospital administration (where the big bucks were and where most of the big bucks went to men at the time), she leapt over to the fast track.

Nimble, she made herself invaluable and soon reached her first benchmark position. She became the Chief Operating Officer—not the top position, but next to the top. She had worked hard and considered herself due for a reward. She had long dreamed of such a treat—a week at a SPA. She made plans to go to a place where she would be catered to, would diet gently to lose the few extra pounds that stress had added to her frame, would exercise, meditate, and read some trashy novels. As she told me about her plans and as her departure approached, I was a bit envious. We were both near forty and she was already in the luxury phase. I knew I could never dream of actually having the experience she was about to have—a fantasy come true. But now, some 15 or so years later, I am pretty sure I have surpassed her. I have had the ultimate spa experience and participated in American Agriculture at the same time. I have been to Wheat Camp.

All it took was the decision my husband and I made to quit

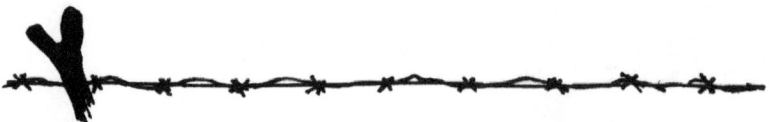

salaried jobs and to farm his family's land to give me the opportunity to find a spa. Perhaps the spa I visited is not the sort for everyone. Wheat Camp (WC for short) isn't advertised on the Internet, but lots of spas are. Let's compare the standard offerings of some of those that have Web sites with WC and you can be the judge.

Several of the ads have some features in common. First, there is the implication, if not the actual statement that the environment is an exclusive one. You might even meet someone famous, incognito of course. There is nothing like high cost to thin out the ranks of participants. Among the establishments I have scouted, the low-end cost is $400 per week for dormitory accommodations; bring your own linens (probably no movie stars there). There is a mid-priced place that may be a bit like Wheat Camp. It's called a boot camp, designed to thin you down and toughen you up in a week. You pay for the privilege of being deprived of food and comfort. The high end is populated with the tonier ones charging more than $5000 per week. They boast that the ratio is at least three staff to each guest and they furnish the fancy bathrobe. (Lots of famous-looking folks at these places.)

Wheat Camp is rather exclusive, also. But, the reason is different. There is no cost to attend. It is our family's annual wheat harvest and is fully staffed by and experienced by my husband, my mother-in-law (who arrives to serve as camp cook) and me. It's not that we intend to exclude anyone; we just have not yet found any takers. (Perhaps after people read this, we will be inundated with applicants.)

Almost all of the spas offer special exercise equipment and instruction in aerobics (both low and high impact). Yoga is also a favorite activity. You can expect to return from the spa more muscular and flexible than when you arrived. The equipment and activity at Wheat Camp accomplish all of the same results and more. For example, we have no need of a stair machine. The ladder to the cab of the combine is five widely-spaced steps from the ground. The climb to the bed of the grain

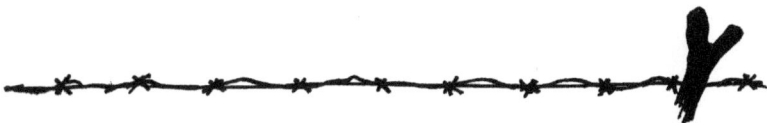

truck must be accomplished with a stepladder combined with a pull-up to hoist one's entire body over the side. Make those circuits several times a day and check the gluteal results. As for the flexibility promised by the postures of traditional hatha yoga, we have none of that. Instead, there are asanas named "swaying stalks of grain," performed bending forward to pluck a stalk to check for moisture; "the rattlesnake," a high backward leap followed by a shout; and "greet the sun while squatting to grease the header," an advanced posture requiring both familiarity with a grease gun and fully functioning knee joints.

Aerobic exercise is that which causes the heart rate to increase, toning the cardiovascular system. Bouncy music, pert instructors and lifting the knees high while performing any of the various routines cutely named "...er-cise" are typical spa approaches to the aerobic state. At WC, all I need to do is pick up the grain scoop and shovel wheat from the front of the grain cart to the auger hole. In only a few minutes, my target heart rate is met! The fact that the ambient temperature is equal to or greater than 95 degrees F speeds the process. Racing to get the tarp cover rolled over the truck bed when a sudden rain shower threatens is also effective. It's either cover the wheat or have the opportunity to cultivate 36,000 pounds of sprouts and sour mash. Gets that heart rate up every time.

Besides the exercise, spas often provide beauty treatments such as manicures, special hair treatments, and facials. They employ an array of materials to open pores, cleanse, exfoliate, soften, and tone every exposed inch of the client. Saunas, special muds, herbs, essential oils, and application techniques with oriental names will pamper you. At Wheat Camp, we have an essential oil, as well. It's 15 W 40. I have applied it to my skin daily and feel well lubricated.

As for the sauna, our equivalent is the combine cab where I climb in each day to vacuum and to replace the duct tape that holds the upholstery in place. (We are small farmers and the combine is old.)

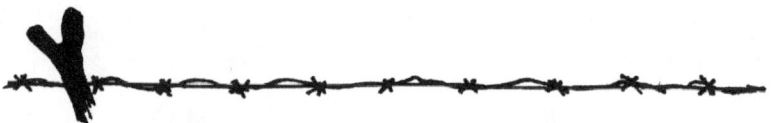

Even without a sauna's heated rocks, the temperature rises rapidly to elicit healing perspiration. Exiting that small chamber into a 25 mph gust of West Texas wind leaves a residue that is not unlike that packaged as Dead Sea Salt. Ah, exfoliation!

Many spas have on-site boutiques that sell clothing suitable to the environment. There is Spandex everywhere, caftans, turbans to cover the hair, and entire lines of footwear—cross trainers, jogging shoes, power-walking shoes, slippers for lounging. My costumes are simpler. Bib overalls, a starched shirt discarded from my husband's cache of dress shirts, and a sports bra with a built-in sweatband are de rigueur. Sturdy high-topped hiking boots and absorbent socks, leather work gloves, and depending on the day, either a large-brimmed straw hat or a "gimme cap" sporting our logo (it says GRAIN AND BEAR IT) complete the outfit. Dressing is finished off with an application of SPF 36 sunscreen to all exposed parts. Our tanning facility is state of the art.

The list of activities at many spas includes lectures. Subjects include stress reduction, nutrition, exercise techniques, women's health, and whatever else is in vogue. As Camp swamper, I receive lectures as well. A swamper is a general assistant who does all manner of menial chores. Instructions in the location of various tools, the proper use of such tools, operation of the transmission in a recalcitrant eight-wheel grain truck, the method for engaging the hydraulic dump apparatus on that truck, etc. are essential to success as a swamper. As a Wheat Camper, my aspiration is to be the *ultimate swamper*.

Food is a big draw for some of the spas. Gourmet fare is advertised, as is low fat nutrition. Wheat Camp's approach to nutrition is a bit different. The concern here is adequate calories to assure necessary energy along with plenty of fluids and comfort foods. This means that chicken fried steak and mashed potatoes are on the menu. That beats anything that relies on radicchio as its matrix.

I could continue. But, I will offer only one other item for

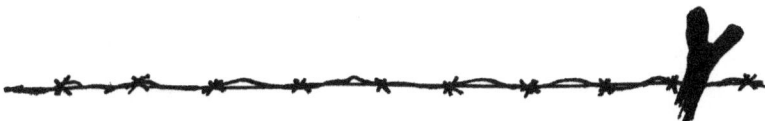

comparison. It is the meditation that spas tout among their wares. Any meditation is good, as far as I am concerned. So, I laud the spas' efforts to encourage a transcendent state for the clients who arrive weary, harried and world worn. Out here on the high plains of Texas, I can enter a trance-like condition without instruction or a special mantra. All I need to do is sit high atop a load of grain or on the combine's fuel tank. I need not close my eyes. The constantly changing scene in the western sky transports me. The sounds of dove and mockingbirds lift my spirit.

The woman whose spa trip I envied told me later that she was bored after two days and was glad that she had taken along some work to do. My guess is that she felt guilty not having evidence of productivity that office paperwork implies. Wheat Camp offers one or two weeks (depends on the weather, equipment breakdowns, and how many acres are planted) of the ultimate in productivity. There's no need to bring paperwork.

Nothing tells you that you are worthy more directly than harvesting what you have sown. Nothing improves health more than delighting in what surrounds us. And nothing leaves me more fit and flexible than my personal version of the spa trip fantasy—Wheat Camp.

—Teddy

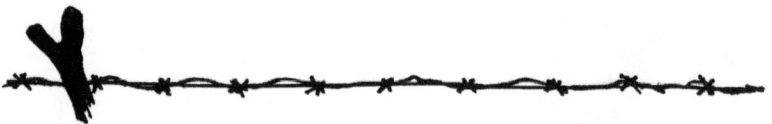

Capsule 82

Horse Sense

*E*very now and then Hollywood gets it right. When the movie "Seabiscuit" was released, I thought to myself that this story, put to book form by Laura Hillenbrand, should be read in all classrooms.

The story chronicles the tale of three men whose lives are intertwined with a horse. The men's ability to trust their instincts and see beyond what was on the outside teaches us all a lesson or two about recognizing potential.

Seabiscuit did not have a commanding presence. He was a small horse. He suffered from Attention Deficit Disorder. He did not trust and sometimes displayed a fierce temper that made many trainers just write him off as belligerent and uncoachable. Enter three very different men at three different times and this horse was transformed to what he was to be: arguably the most instinctive winner in horseracing history. It's also possible that Seabiscuit wasn't transformed. He had possessed the qualities needed to win from the start.

"Horses stay the same from the day they are born until the day they die...they are only changed by the way people treat them." Trainer Tom Smith nailed it. It really is horse sense to grasp that animals, or people, always have within them what it takes.

Animals and people interact all the time on farms and ranches. Almost anyone who has grown up around those settings has developed

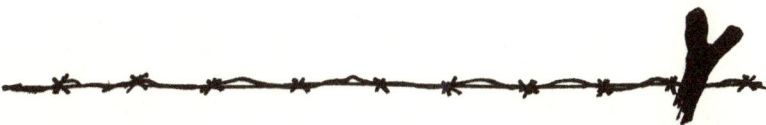

a knack for knowing and loving the creatures that serve both as companions and fellow workers. The sheep dogs, the horses, the barn cats, or the show animals become like family.

I have often found it ironic, though, that people often treat people with far less respect. If the lessons learned in the country could transfer to human relationships, it's safe to say that a lot of psychologists would have a lot fewer appointments.

Rural people should have a heads up on getting along with people and recognizing potential. They do it every day in their work—with their animals, their crops, their herds of cattle. They automatically look for prospects, nurture the object to bring about results, and have trained eyes to spot a winner. Why can't that be done with looking at children or spouses? What is it that prevents people from nurturing people the way they do their bird dogs?

Many years before a quiet horse trainer spoke those words about horses, the German philosopher, Goethe, practically said the same thing about people:

"Treat people as if they were what they ought to be, and you help them to become what they are capable of becoming."

We would all benefit from learning to see more than meets the eye. Tom Howard also said, "Learn your horse. Each one is an individual, and once you penetrate his mind and heart, you can often work wonders."

It makes sense, doesn't it?

—Sue Jane

 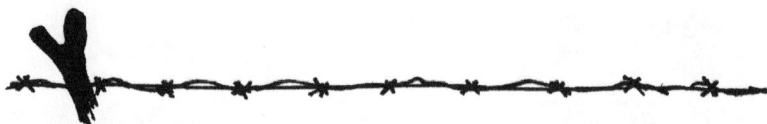

Capsule 83

Friday Nights in the Fall

*P*ick-up trucks surround the field, but the men in the community stand along the chain link fence just yards from the chalk lines. If the weather is bad, the women and children will sometimes sit in the vehicles. Most of the time, however, they pack the stands, with just enough room left for the pep squad and perhaps a small band. It's Friday night in September, and that means football in even the smallest of communities.

Even where high school enrollment is fewer than 50 students, football is still a part of the American dream for boys. Thanks to the ingenuity of a Nebraska man in 1933, six-man football has allowed many athletes in smaller schools to participate in a sport seen as a rite of passage.

Dr. Stephen Epler coached at Chester High School in the 1930s. Like many small schools, Chester struggled to field a team of at least 11 to play football. The solution was simple in Epler's mind—invent a game where fewer boys could play but keep the rules of football the same.

He settled on six so as to keep the same number of ends on either side of the center. The quarterback had one other blocker with an additional running back or wide receiver.

With just six guys on either side of the ball, the game is usually highlighted by a lot of scoring. It is not unusual for Saturday morning sports pages to report games with scores like 56–40 or 68–32. In six-man

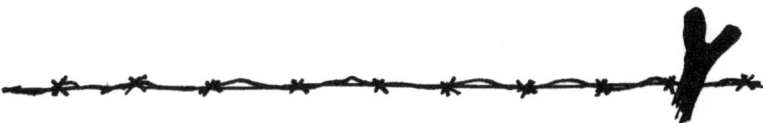

football, offense wins games. If a defensive-minded coach happens to be in charge, that's just icing on the cake.

Besides the fact that small schools can compete in the sport of football, this modified game is also a boon to the smaller player. Guys who wouldn't be able to make a team in a larger school know they have a chance on six-man teams, and not just because of the diminished enrollment. Physical size in a player may be more crucial in an 11-man system, but speed and quickness are rewarded on the six-man playing field. Some of the best players on a six-man field are well under six feet tall and weigh less than 170 lbs.

Speaking of the playing field, there are some interesting differences in the dimensions of the field. Rather than 100 x 50 (length and width), the six-man football field is 80 yards in length and only 40 yards wide.

Teams have the regular four downs to get a first down, but they must advance the ball fifteen yards instead of ten. Touchdowns are six points, but extra points differ due to the ease with which a kick can be blocked on an extra point attempt. If the kick is successful, the offense gets two points. If the offense runs or throws for the extra point after the touchdown, they are awarded only one point.

The degree of difficulty is also noted in the points awarded to a field goal which is four—with only three people to block against six defenders, Epler believed that a kick through the uprights warranted such a change in the scoring system from the traditional 11-man rules.

In the 70 years since its debut, six-man football has allowed many boys from farm and ranch backgrounds the opportunity to participate other sports beside basketball or track. Some boys who travel the rodeo circuit view six-man football as a natural extension of their athletic pursuits because of some similarities between the two.

For example, many tackles in six-man ball are open field, a move similar to ones cowboys make when trying to wrestle down a steer.

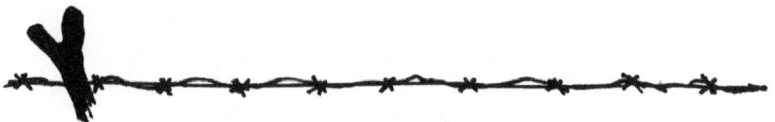

Roping, which includes heading and heeling, is a perfect analogy for what a defender does on the solo tackles in six-man football—he may tackle high while his teammate goes for the legs.

Many of the men in the small communities move from cotton rows to fence rows on Friday night. They are extended versions of the armchair quarterback as they chew and dip and cuss their way through four quarters of football. The only difference is that the players they watch are their sons, their grandsons, their nephews, and maybe the young man that drives a tractor for them in the summer.

Six-man football is not just a sport in a small town. It is a community event, and from miles around, the citizens of that community drive to support the concession stand, the band, the pep squad, and of course, the six men who line up to play the same fundamental game the Dallas Cowboys play on Sunday.

—Sue Jane

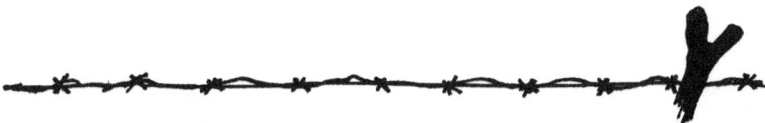

Capsule 84

The Stock Show Zone—Episode XXII Trading Spaces

Setting: a showbarn in Small Town, USA, one week before the county livestock show

Host: Vocational Ag. Instructor Buddy Ray Wallace and his FFA children, Kate and Tyler Wallace

Scene: 14-year old Kate, owner of two show lambs named Wilma and Betty, exchanges animals with her 17-year-old brother Tyler, who has two Durocs named Fred and Barney. Each sibling must conduct extreme makeovers on the animals, preparing them for the upcoming county stock show. They must also re-do the holding pens for the stock. Their father, Buddy Ray, will serve as guide and referee.

Kate: "Dad, how much money are you going to give me to work with?"

Buddy Ray (Dad): "Sugar, you can have as much as you need."

Tyler: "How about me, Pop?"

Buddy Ray: "Son, you get exactly one hundred forty six dollars and thirty-two cents. Not a dime more. And don't talk back to me."

Tyler: "Dad..."

Buddy Ray: "Okay. Now you're down to one hundred ten dollars and thirty-two cents."

Kate: "Oh, my gosh, this is going to be so much fun. Tyler, I guarantee

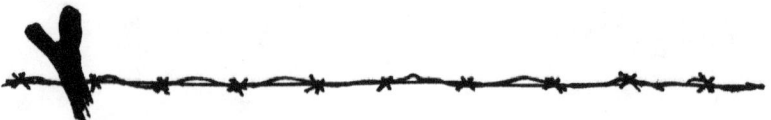

Barney and Fred are going to win the stock show after I get through with them."

Tyler: "Kate, if they do, it's because I have taken care of them for six months."

Kate: "What's to take care of? Everyone knows that of all the stock show animals, the hogs are the easiest. They eat, they sleep, they walk around a little. Just like you."

Tyler: "Yeah, and your dumb sheep have to be fed daily because they aren't smart enough to do a self-feeder."

Kate: "So? At least they have pretty wool to work with."

Tyler (aside): "Not for long...hee, hee, hee.

Scene Change: Two days before the stock show. A scream is heard from the show barn. Junior Livestock Association Members, volunteers, concerned parents, and nosey community members with nothing better to do come running in the direction of the cry.

Kate (distraught and in need of a gentle slap across the face): "My little woolen babies! Oh, my little sweet Southdowns—what did he do to you? Daddy!"

Mr. Holmes (sheep show superintendent): "Honey, it will be okay. We'll just enter them in a different category."

Mrs. York (concerned parent): "Now don't you fret, Hon. That rainbow look is really popular this year."

Mr. Limbaugh (nosey community member): "Yeah, on snowcones."

Buddy Ray: "Tyler! Kate, darling, please don't cry. I'll handle this after I handle your brother."

(Meanwhile, another cry is heard from another part of the showbarn. This one is even shriller and more distraught.)

Tyler: "No, not fuchsia!"

Buddy Ray: "What's wrong with you?" (Buddy Ray notices that Fred and

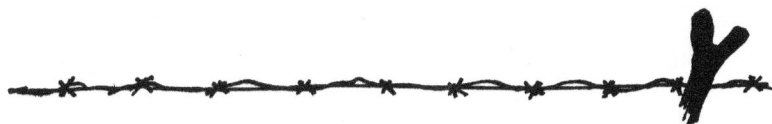

Barney, hanging from the rafters, have been manicured, pedicured, and cured.)

Tyler: "Golly, Dad, why did she have to go and use that color?!"
Buddy Ray: "You've got a point, son. At least she stayed within the lines. Kate!!"

(With a sheepish look, Kate, consoled by Mrs. York and Mrs. Smith, approaches her dad and brother. The three embrace and cry hysterically. Mr. Limbaugh gets sick and throws up. Fortunately, one of the stray cats in the showbarn is available for janitorial duty. The crowd disperses in order for the family unit to deal with their dysfunctional moment.)

Buddy Ray (wiping away the tears with his bandana): "Kids, we have exactly four hours until the swine show. Tomorrow morning is the lamb show. You know what we have to do."
Kate: "I guess that science project paid off after all, Dad."
Tyler: "Easy for you to say, Kate. What am I supposed to do, Dad?"
Buddy Ray: "Go help her load the clones!"

(Tyler turns and shuffles out of the showbarn, taking one last look at his cured hams and vowing to get revenge.)

Tyler: "Load the clones, my foot. I made an A on my science project, too. Time to bring out the laser shears."

Narrator: Small town USA. The community stock show. Moments like this—are they real? Or, is it only the stock show zone?

—Sue Jane

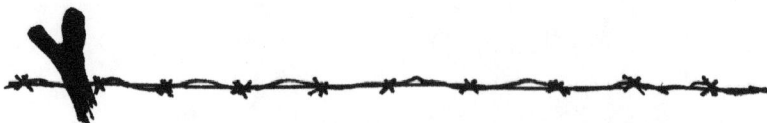

Capsule 85

Support Your Local EMT

 M y mom says I once stuck rocks up my nose—completely filled both nostrils. At least Mom could see them and respond quickly. When she couldn't get them out herself, she had to drive me 35 miles to the hospital. That was 1959.

First response is critical with most emergencies, though my attempt at a Guinness record hardly qualified as a major emergency. It is especially important in rural areas where medical treatment is usually miles and many minutes away.

Since 1975 when laws gave license to rural emergency medical technicians (EMT), first response now is often provided by someone other than a parent. Rural emergency medical technicians not only offer a vital link to larger hospitals, they do it voluntarily in most cases.

To become an EMT requires 140 classroom, 32 hours of hospital emergency room observation, and 32 hours of ambulance runs. This is time spent after they have worked a full day on the farm or ranch or another job in the county. The training may or may not be funded by a county entity; if not, the expense for books, labs, and hours is out of pocket.

In the county where I live, the local EMT service operates two ambulances, both secured as a result of grants written by the local EMT director. In another rare but fortunate situation, our county's seven

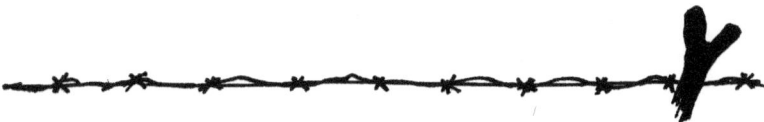

personnel are all paramedics. Their training has extended well beyond the basic EMT level.

In Borden County, some 80% of dispatches are personal. In other words, the residents call a local number or the sheriff's office. The option of 911 now exists, but those calls are re-routed. The first responder may just be down the farm-to-market road and better yet, a neighbor who knows the victim(s). That makes it easier to make the call direct and for the help to be immediate and personal.

With their vested interest, EMTs and paramedics in rural areas accept calls in the middle of the night, attend the local athletic events, and help strangers driving through the county on major highways. Theirs is a 24-hour shift, without rotation.

Critical shortages exist in some counties. Despite free ambulance service in many rural areas, residents are still taking the efforts of these volunteer medical technicians for granted. Monetary donations help the cause, but these volunteers need helping hands.

Consider making an investment of money and time to a cause that perhaps will buy time for those in need of emergency treatment. Support your local EMTs. A life saved may be your own.

—Sue Jane

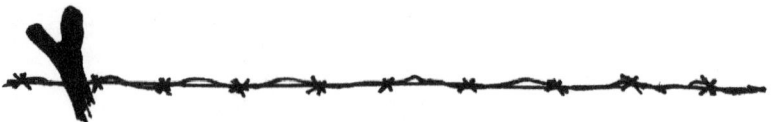

Capsule 86

A Real Gift

Reminiscing—recalling and retelling occurrences in one's past—is not the exclusive province of the elderly. You can confirm that by listening to conversations at a class reunion or family gathering.

Here's one I heard. "I remember that time we all loaded into Rodney's old Ford and drove out to that abandoned house," Jimmy starts. "Oh yeah," Charlie interrupts, "and three of us hid upstairs while everyone else was looking around downstairs." Not to be outdone, Jimmy takes up again, "And then we jumped out to scare them when the girls came up the stairs. Everyone started screaming except you (pointing to one of the girls-grown-older). And you just said 'I knew it was Gary. I could smell his Aqua Velva.'"

A story of a shared experience may have different meaning to each participant, from "I loved that old Ford" to "you were a little different from the rest of the girls" or "did I really wear that much Aqua Velva?" Each meaning prompts thoughts about who we were and who we have become.

Gerontologists say that reminiscing has value for all of us, but can be particularly beneficial as a person ages. Rather than being a symptom of "living in the past," reminiscence reflects a natural process of life review. Their research suggests that memories surface throughout life, along with associated emotions. But, as one ages, there may be

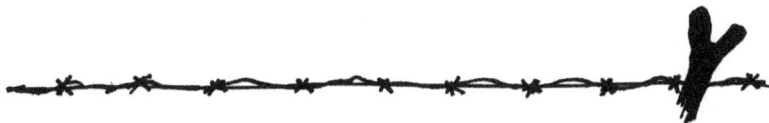

fewer distractions and the person may expend less effort to prevent focusing on those memories. As a result, as we age, recall of the past can become quite vivid. And, as with eyewitness accounts of any event, different individuals' memories of the same event may vary.

Consider how a birthday party might be recalled by the honoree, a guest and the hostess. One remembers receiving a longed-for gift of a bicycle, another recalls the backyard swing set breaking under the weight of too many guests on the see-saw, and mom visualizes the mess on her new carpet.

For each one, his or her own memory is the truth of the event. That story may be relegated to the memory as an isolated occurrence, without reflection or much meaning. Or a memory reflected upon and joined with others can become part of a person's notion of who they are. That might be, "Almost everything I've ever wished for, I've received." Or, "I was too fat, even then, or that swing set wouldn't have broken when I got on." The mother's view might be "I've always had to clean up after everyone else."

The lifelong process of reminiscing, as a part of knowing ourselves, can become more important in late life. It can help bring serenity, wisdom, or help resolve long-held conflicts through acceptance. Reminiscing can also prompt sadness, anger, and grieving. Regardless, no emotion is, in itself, bad for us. To feel is human. What is not good for us is to hold back emotion (happy, sad or in between) or to ignore, without reflection, memories that prompt the emotion.

Unfortunately, as a person ages, there often are fewer people with whom to share memories. Daily life consumes the interest of younger family members and the age mates of the elderly become fewer with each year.

But, there is a helpful, healthful gift you can give to an aging person. You can think of it as a game. In some elder care facilities it's called "Reminiscence Therapy." Groups meet with a staff member who

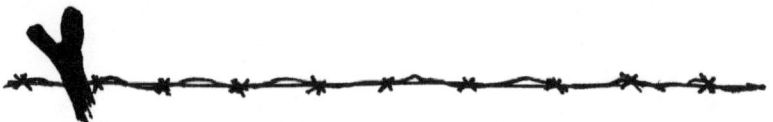

brings up topics to prompt reminiscing. An object, such as washboard, is shown to the group or a newspaper account of major event like the bombing of Pearl Harbor is read. Participants are then encouraged to tell their related memories.

But, if you decide to "give this gift", you don't need a group. In fact, the best reminiscing happens when a person has the undivided attention of one other person whose main function is to just listen. You can encourage the person to get started in the same way you might start any visit, just say why you came by. "I was thinking that you might have some interesting stories to tell about (fill in the blank) and I wondered if you have time to visit some about that today." You can encourage with comments like, "What else was happening then? Who was there? Looks like it makes you happy to remember that. Crying's okay when you feel sad."

There is no need to correct facts or dates or to offer judgments about what is remembered. These are memories. The events are in the past. But, it can be useful to assure the person that whatever they tell you will not repeat to anyone. Of course, if you promise that, you must mean it.

You are not "doing therapy" but the reminiscence may be therapeutic. That's a real gift.

—Teddy

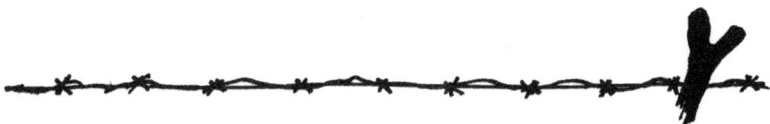

Capsule 87

Nostalgia

*...telling a poet not to look for connections is like telling a
farmer not to look at the rain gauge after a storm.*
—Kathleen Norris, *Dakota: A Spiritual Geography*

*M*y dad's fascination with trains has passed down to me. He grew up in Texarkana and spent many an hour watching the trains at the city's hub station. This was entertainment for a young boy in the 1930s.

The Roscoe, Snyder & Pacific Railroad near US Highway 84 came through my small town. I loved to count the cars and my older brother loved to disrupt my counting by any devious means possible. The argument would start something like this:

Me: "forty-two, forty-three, forty-four, forty-five..."
Big Brother (with horns and a forked tail): "Hey, did I tell you that I made a seventy-six on a math test, Dad? Or was that a sixty-seven? Anyway, my average is now seventy-two which is considerably higher than the sixty-four I had last semester."

Needless to say, it would take me awhile to get back on track. I was persistent, though, because I knew it would all add up to the symbol of all symbols, the red caboose.

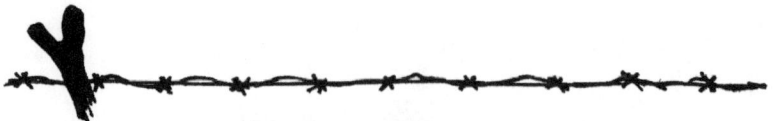

Not long ago when I was driving a lonely stretch of rural road, a train's passing had the same effect as it had 35 years earlier. I wanted to call my brother on his cell phone and boast about the 56 cars counted without having to start over. Instead of being nostalgic about those station wagon quarrels, I became nostalgic about something I did not see. There was no red caboose at the end of the train.

Cabooses originally were built to protect the crew's cooking fires. Later they became the crew's accommodations. Train trips without stops used to be longer, so the necessity of having such accommodations was evident. Today, the trains that are still in service have shorter routes. The crew won't be cooking and usually won't be staying in what was once called the "way car" or the "shanty."

The noticeable void for me that day, though, was the realization that my children have missed out on the nostalgic symbols of the railcar that brought up the rear. Red cabooses were symbols of anticipation at the end of my counting, symbols of a man wearing a conductor's cap waving out the window at children waving back from a 1966 yellow station wagon, symbols of campaign speeches in presidential election years. Cabooses were closure. Whenever I saw the caboose, I knew I could go back to reading a book or slapping my brother.

Perhaps my parents noticed when I was a child that I grew up without a front porch swing. My generation also missed out on Saturday evening radio shows. The list could be endless. That's why nostalgia is so important. If we do not appreciate it, the list will end.

Nostalgia is nothing but a connector of the past to the present. Certainly some things are better left in the past—like hand crank ice cream makers—but the memories made around that crank should not be, pardon the expression, frozen in time.

—Sue Jane

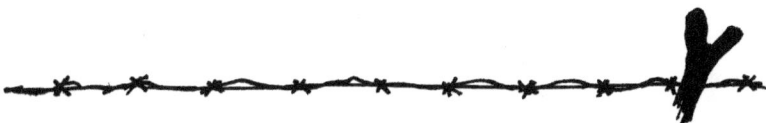

Capsule 88

Highway 6

*T*here's nothing on this stretch of road.

Exactly, I thought, pleased that I had chosen this route to drive from my small town in West Texas to Waco to watch a ballgame.

My travel companions—one daughter and some teenage friends—had yet to learn to appreciate what was obvious to me. Nothing is good sometimes. Especially when the landscape is as lovely as it is in late fall or during spring rains on Texas Highway 6.

Now, by nothing, I don't mean to imply that little towns like Gorman or Hico or DeLeon or Meridian have nothing to offer. On the contrary, they have some of the quaintest shops in Texas. There are bookstores, hunting supply depots, Norwegian bakeries, Czech bakeries, and some great convenience stores with clean restrooms and lots of peanut patties. (This is peanut country, too!) Dublin, another small spot on the map, is even the home of what is probably most Texans' preferred beverage, Dr. Pepper.

By nothing, I simply mean that the landscape remains just that, landscape. Land can be seen. Country homes are visible. Cattle and sheep and goats roam the pastures. There is no thing that is taking away from nature. And I, for one, like that a lot.

Some small towns are succumbing to a blitz of marketing that is bringing superstores to their area. Where the small grocery store or

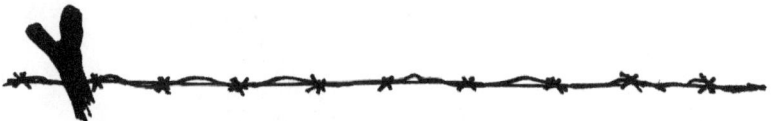

specialty shops were the norm, some small towns on interstate highways now have the "convenience" of shopping large, just like the city folks do. Driving down an interstate is like driving on one extended big city boulevard, at times. It all runs together. Not on Highway 6.

The traffic is busy but not stifling. Pickup trucks and hay haulers are common sights. Old folks driving those big Buicks don't mind getting on this road because they know they probably won't get plowed over by someone in a big hurry. Seldom are people in a hurry on this stretch of road. I know at least that I never am. It's a beauty, and I like to take my time soaking in the elms and oaks and pecans.

Cattle crossings come every few hundred yards. Small farms are noticeable from just off the highway; the larger ones are located farther back from the road. The livestock that graze on these farms are fat and happy. This part of the state usually receives steady rainfall to keep stock tanks full and fields green.

It occurs to me that people who live in cities don't get to point out their car windows and say to their small children, "See the cows! What do the cows say?" Their children have to learn all of that on some Mattel Spin and Say game or on a big wooden puzzle. My girls got to learn it first hand. I remind my daughter of that on this particular trip. She just rolls her eyes, but I know she understands. She'll do the same thing someday with her kids.

Have you found a road like Highway 6 in your state? Perhaps yours is one of the farms or ranches that adjoins a beautiful stretch of pavement like this one. But part of the beauty of finding a wonderful road like this is that it's away from home, but seems like home. So if you search for your own "Highway 6," bear that in mind.

Many of the things that attract me to Highway 6 are the same things I have at home; six-man football games, special celebrations, local one-of-a-kind attractions. But the combination of familiarity and different locale creates a powerful attraction, made even more attractive by the

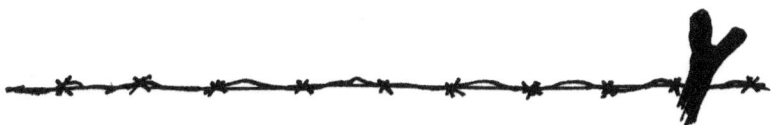

absence of hustle, bustle, and metropolitan sameness.

Someday I'm going to stop in Gorman on a Friday night for a six-man football game. Another time I'll make a trip for the Peanut Festival at DeLeon or see if I can't get a gig as a food judge at the county fair. I'll top it off with a six-pack of 100% Dr. Pepper. (Locals know that Dublin Dr. Pepper has lots more kick than the kind you buy in other convenience stores across the country because it's made with 100% pure cane sugar.)

I'm sure many articles have appeared about Highway 6, in numerous publications, written by people who really are journalists. In those you can find the details of restaurants, lodgings, and bed and breakfast places. That's fine. Those writers get paid to travel and write about what they see.

I'm just a traveler who likes to write, and all I know is that this winding road between Eastland and Waco has wound itself around my heart for the simple reason that it's naturally pleasing to the eye. I can't wait to get on that road again.

—Sue Jane

Capsule 89

You Produce A Precious Commodity

*I*f there is a group of people who understand change and uncertainty, it is those in agriculture. A farm or ranch woman will be the first to point out that nothing at all is ever the same from one day to the next. Plants grow and die, livestock move through stages of development, the land changes with the weather, and the people we know affect and are affected by the land, the elements, their crops and livestock, and one another while passing through the stages of their lives. When a person so acutely aware of constant change hears what has been uttered so often since September 11, 2001, "Nothing will ever be the same," their first response may be a very realistic one: "Nothing *is ever* the same from one day to the next."

That perspective, realism based on being intimately connected to the cycles of life, can be the basis for an important commodity in times of crisis. That commodity is *hope.*

Crisis, a condition of major upheaval, is change. It is change that is vast and/or unanticipated and for which usual methods of coping seem inadequate. National crisis becomes personal crisis whenever individuals feel that they may be affected personally. Terrorist acts within our country make threat feel personal. Any threat or personal uncertainty can affect our mental health and our whole being. In the long term, those negative

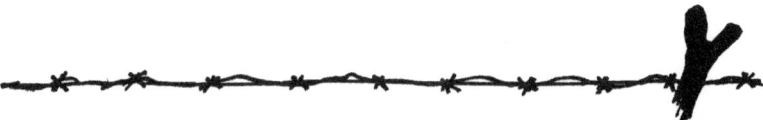

effects can be as destructive as the very direct physical consequences of terrorist acts.

Farmers and ranchers, perhaps more than many other people, have developed over generations the skills to cope with crises. These same skills that have meant personal and group survival through other crises can be applied to new crises as they arise. The most basic of those coping skills is identifying what we can affect and that over which we have no control. We cannot control the weather but we can decide when to plow or plant. We have little direct control over market prices but we can decide whether or when to sell livestock. We have little or no control over the acts of individual terrorists but we can choose to be aware of appropriate personal protective measures and to increase personal vigilance.

And after we have sorted the controllable from that which we cannot change, we can focus on continuing—on proceeding with working, eating, sleeping, and caring for ourselves and for those around us. Those are the most basic requirements of life and those over which we have the greatest control.

Another coping skill is anxiety reduction. Stress management reduces anxiety. This is a high priority because of the numerous negative physical, mental, and spiritual problems created when anxiety is high. Start by paying attention only to accurate information, not rumor, opinion, or supposition. Take care to sort between fact and all the rest and grant yourself the peace of retreating from "news" for at least several hours each day. Instead of listening to phone-in radio programs or the endless repeats of hourly TV news and market reports, practice simple calming techniques such as slow deep breathing and conscious muscle relaxation several times each day. Simple as that seems, it does reduce anxiety.

Helping those around you is beneficial both to them and to you. Teach them what you know about managing anxiety and stress and you are reinforcing those lessons for yourself. Children, in particular, may

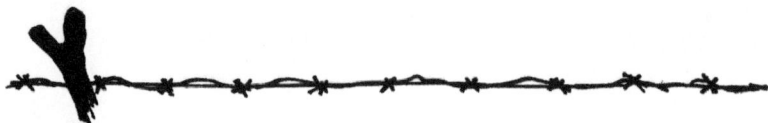

need an opportunity to talk about their anxiety and to be guided toward a hopeful outlook. While they may not directly express anxiety, you may notice differences in behavior such as clinginess in young children or irritability or withdrawal in an older child. Encourage them to ask questions and be factual and truthful in your answers. When you do not have facts to answer their questions, show them how to use their abilities to think, reason and gather information to find those answers. For example, a personal demonstration of how to use the atlas to find the distance from your home to the Middle East is both supportive and educational. Talk about the fact that it natural and intelligent to be afraid when danger is present. Explain in examples they can relate to. Demonstrate for them your own hopefulness and they will learn it from you.

People in agriculture produce the commodities that help make our country run. People in agriculture have always been notable for their characteristic ability to endure and to continue in the face of adversity of all sorts. That can only be based on the fact that among the commodities you produce, one of the most precious is hope.

—Teddy

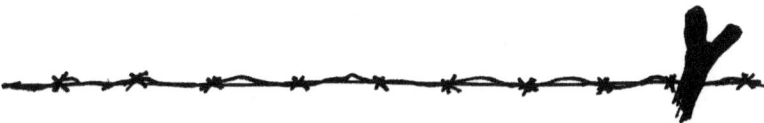

Capsule 90

Hard Times And How To Help

Standing at the cemetery in the West Texas wind, I realized that attending three funerals in one month as I have recently gives a person more than the usual number of things to reflect on. Among those things I have pondered since that time is the effect of grief on a person's health. While grief dealt with poorly can lead to lingering depression, the natural sadness and ambivalence that accompanies a loss is not necessarily unhealthy. Humans grieve all sorts of losses, not only the loss of friends or loved ones taken by death. For some, loss of function, such as results from chronic illnesses is cause for grief. For others, loss of a job or loss of status prompts the same feelings. In fact, any loss, of a person, an object or in a person's estimate of themselves is a natural cause for grief. These are hard times for those who grieve and we want to help.

Healthy responses to grief are those that allow and encourage a person to recognize all the emotions that they are feeling and to express them. That sounds simple, but putting the prescription in action is not so simple. Sadness, anger, fear or anxiety, even relief, may all crowd together. The person grieving may feel quite out of control of his or her emotions. That's very different than the composed way that most of us try to present ourselves to the world. But, feeling these emotions is *not* illness. Rather, it is quite human. The health—promoting thing to do is

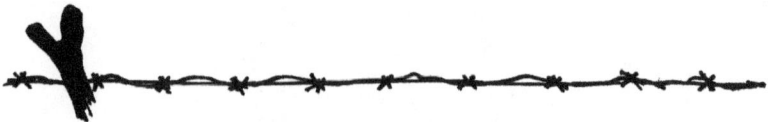

to help ourselves or others to go through the process of grieving rather than to run from or suppress the emotions. Suppressed emotion is a lot like steam—it cannot be held in its original container as it is generated by the heat and boiling water. It has to have an outlet and will find one, either healthy or unhealthy.

Over time, some rituals have developed, differing from one culture to another, that provide a person opportunity to express some of the emotion. These rituals, such as funerals, encourage us to cry, to remember, to say goodbye. For those with certain religious beliefs, these occasions and their religious significance are an important source of comfort.

Retirement dinners are another ritual for much the same purpose. Unfortunately, we do not have rituals to help us deal with some other important losses such as damage to our estimates of ourselves. The cultures we live in do not yet have ceremonies to mark bankruptcies or divorces.

While the ritual events are useful, they do not mark the end of grieving. Nor is it realistic to expect that people can "pull themselves together" and finish their grieving in a day or two. Grieving takes time and it takes energy.

Well-meaning friends and family have the potential to be the greatest help to a person who is grieving. I qualify that by the phrase "have the potential" because those same well-intentioned people can make things worse just as easily. An example—giving advice to the grieving person to get medication right away to keep from feeling sad or to discourage crying is *not* a way to help the expression of emotion. It would be far better to simply sit quietly and pass the tissues to one who needs to cry. A caring presence does not have to include doing anything more than caring and taking the time to be present.

Besides tears, words are an excellent way to express emotion. Some are more skilled than others at getting a person to talk—about

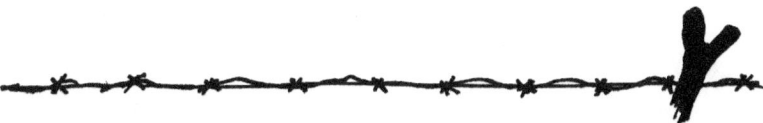

their feelings—rather than just about the ordinary topics of conversation. Many of us are cautious about speaking of our emotions to others. We have to be encouraged to do it. Better yet, we need to be assured confidentiality when we do. "It might help to talk about the feelings you have been having. If you would like to do that, I can promise to keep our conversation just between us." That is one type of encouragement. Or, if your history with the grieving person makes confidentiality a guarantee, you might just say, "This must be a really confusing time, all kinds of feelings all jumbled together. I would be happy to just listen if you would like to talk about that." It is not very helpful to offer "look on the bright side" comments or to use the visit as an opportunity to recount similar experiences of your own, in detail. And, while I have no scientific evidence to support this, I believe that phone conversations take second place to face-to-face visits for such purposes.

Another comfort is food. Bringing a meal or some special treat, not just on funeral day, but on occasion in the weeks or months following a loss can symbolize caring.

Do what you can. Losses are hard times and you can help.

—Teddy

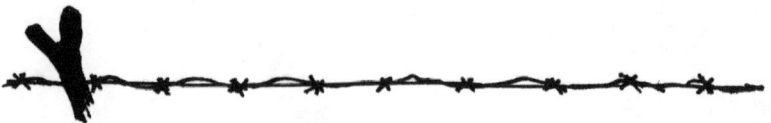

Capsule 91

Reading Between the Lines

A September 1931 bank statement, checks written in pencil, drafted on the Rotan National Bank in Rotan, Texas, told a story of financial responsibility and pride. One could also infer from these few yellowed pieces of paper that grief did not prevent my grandmother from being practical in how she managed her money.

Life insurance was a luxury during the Depression decade. There were far more tangible matters to tend to, like food, shelter, and clothing. For some reason, though, my grandparents chose to buy life insurance and to scrape together the money to make the monthly premium payments.

The ironic thing about life insurance is that you hope you never have to cash in your chips. You realize that paying a premium is pretty much money thrown away unless someone dies. How assuring is that?

Only three months after a baby (my mother) was born in April, my grandfather died from complications after being gassed while cleaning out a well on the family farm. His sons (my two uncles), ages 5 and 10, were with him along with my grandfather's brother. Uncle Preston and Uncle Clifton had to run to a neighbor's house to get help. Grandfather was revived and was carried to the hospital in Stamford some 45 miles away, but he died the next day.

Grandmother had lost her husband, her best friend, and the father to her five children, all of whom now were dependent on her—a woman

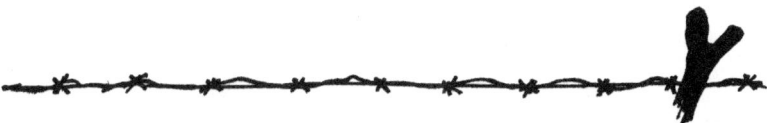

at the age of 41—to provide during the country's bleakest economic times, the Depression.

And provide she did.

The bank statement that came in September 1931 following the August accident shows that Grandmother took the two life insurance checks and immediately made some prudent decisions. She could have indulged her grief as people often do today with material things such as travel, new clothes, and a vehicle. Grandmother paid bills. She paid off the note on the farm. She paid debts owed to family members from whom Grandfather had borrowed. She used some to help her own mother who had financial need.

She was now the manager, and if women were valued then in such corporate positions as they are now, Grandmother easily would have been a CEO. But all she wanted was the farm and for her children to be able to stay together—she knew her chances of that happening were based on her ability to hold on to the land and prove she could manage the farm.

She lived for 25 more years after, passing away when my mother was just four months shy of giving birth to me. No doubt working a farm alone took its toll. She was only 66 at the time of her death.

Obviously, Grandmother succeeded in the two things she wanted more than anything after Grandfather died. The farm (some 220 acres in Fisher County) remains in our family today, and her five children made sure the family bond meant something even though they lived in Washington, Texas, and Virginia. Her grandchildren grew up knowing their aunts and uncles by more than just their names. They, along with her great-grandchildren, still gather every two years for a McCleskey reunion.

Grandmother insured all of this, with a policy on paper and a policy in her heart that family mattered most.

—Sue Jane

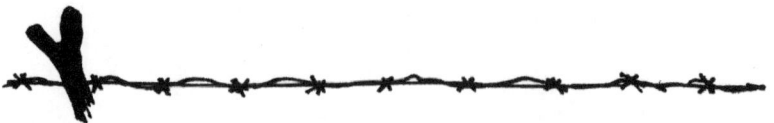

Capsule 92

A Quilt Made Of Love

*T*he death of a schoolteacher in a small town affects many. They include the classes of school children whom she taught, the co-workers she saw daily, and the members of the community with whom she served in many varied roles, from stock show mentor to cheerleader sponsor.

But none feel the loss in quite the same way as her own children, with whom she traveled to many a rodeo, stock show, and ball game in her favorite "job" of all—mom.

A Eulogy for Their Mother

Their mother was not the thread that held them together.
She was the seamstress, the maker of their quilt—and what a
beautiful pattern she created in the three of them.
And in her work, she labored with threads unique to her
that made her quilt what it was.
She used the threads of devotion.
This person in their lives whose loss they now grieve—and rightfully
so—was devoted to her children—to their interests, to their well
being, to their education, to their triumphs, and a devoted presence
in their struggles—a devotion that comes instinctively from a
mother's heart.
She used the threads of joy.
Few people had as beautiful and captivating a smile as their mother did.

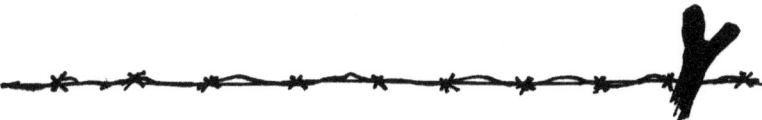

And nothing, no one gave her as great a reason to smile,
as did her children.
Throughout the years of athletics and cheerleading and academic
and musical accomplishments, during the AJRA and stock show
years, their mother was there to share those fun times with them.
It is what she lived for. And, after the three of them were gone from
Borden County Schools, she transferred her joy to the children she
taught. Mother became Mrs. Key, and as any good teacher will do,
she loved her school children with a similar joy.
She used the threads of diligence.
Her labors at home and at school were marked by the drive to do
them well. She organized and agonized over details to make things
work right, and this drive for perfection was not one of an obsessive-
compulsive nature—it was a reflection of someone doing her best
because that is what one is supposed to do.
And finally, their mother used the thread that tied
everything together—love,
a word that is easily spoken and spoken of, but one that is hard to get
right in so many relationships. Never did she waver in the love she
had for the three of them The sweetest words in her vocabulary were
Brice, Ralynn, and Grant. Her success as a person can now be
measured not by how wonderfully she always dressed—and she
did—or how courageously she fought this disease—and she did.
Her success is now seen in them:
In Brice, as a husband and father.
In Ralynn, as a wife, a mother, a teacher.
And in Grant, as a young man finishing college
with a promising future.
The three of them now as brothers and sister will use devotion, joy,
diligence and love to hold their family together in the years to come.
The seamstress is no longer with them, but they can wrap themselves
in her quilt. It is her legacy to them and will warm their broken
hearts until they see her in another time, another place.

—Sue Jane

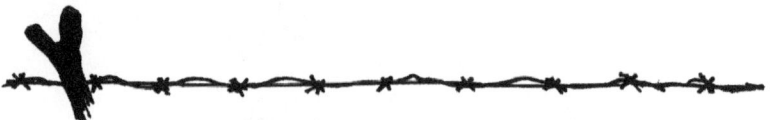

Capsule 93

More Than The Price Of Admission

Both admission and coffee were free that day. And it was a perfect day as far as I was concerned—vivid blue sky , temperature 20 degrees, several inches of snow frozen crunchy overnight. The auction lot was filled with equipment. Spray rigs on trailers, 38-inch tractor tires, cotton strippers, vintage bobtail grain trucks, field cultivators with their "arms" folded, planters, listers, out-of-work mold board plows, many items the names of which I do not know, one combine (comes with two headers), and several tractors could have meant anything. Perhaps their sale was the next step toward retirement for an older farmer. Another person's equipment may have been for sale in order to satisfy debts. For others, the auction was the opportunity to buy at bargain prices. For me, this was an educational experience, a field trip.

I thought that I was attending my first farm sale to see how it was done and to learn more about farm equipment. The camera around my neck was a perfect costume. It prompted folks to talk to me by making them curious. Those conversations and the view I had through the lens taught me more than I expected that day. Auction and equipment were only a part of what was happening. The rest was Health Promotion and Disease Prevention in one of its best forms, face-to-face human interaction.

What can attending an auction remedy or prevent? Social

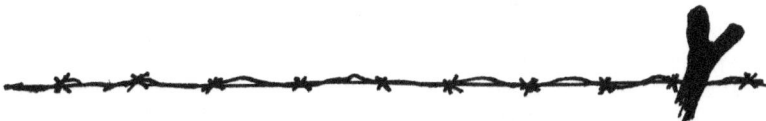

isolation. Rural dwellers are not alone in their potential to become isolated. Anyone who has reduced contact with other humans, by choice or by circumstance, can suffer the results of isolation. A very common result is depression. That depression may be mild, sufficient to reduce the joy of each day and to magnify every ache and pain to giant proportions but not enough for others to notice. Or, the depression may be more severe, producing more profound distress of body, mind, and spirit.

Even if one does not suffer depression, isolation reduces the buffers and support that a person needs to cope with stress and crises when they occur. A clear example of the result of this need for social support to help in coping is that the incidence of family violence is high in remote areas.

We all differ in the amount of social support and interaction that we like or feel we need. But, even the most rugged individualists would probably agree that total isolation from social interaction is not desirable. Social isolation can occur anywhere. One can choose not to participate in group activities, to eliminate contact with family, and to talk only to their cats in the city as easily as in a rural area. Children grow up and leave home, spouses die, friends move away from everyone, no matter where we live. As we age, potential for those situations that can isolate us increase. This is true regardless of location.

But, the fact that a rural person lives 20 miles from town and 10 miles from the nearest neighbor makes it much easier to have isolation become a problem. The same features that are attractive to some of us—space to roam, land to tend, minimum traffic, no noise, and fewer people—also create a larger risk for isolation's negative effects.

People fool themselves if they believe that if they watch TV, they have reduced their isolation. Being aware of the news of the day does not eliminate social isolation. And keeping up with the activities of

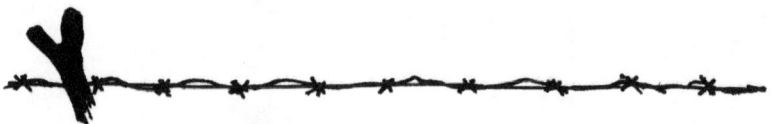

family and acquaintances by telephone is not the same as face-to-face interaction. Our stories are best told in person.

As the morning warmed up and the snow gave way to mud, the men at the sale moved around, looking at equipment and striking up conversations. Some of them had come from 100 or more miles away. Several visited with me. One talked about a health problem. Another reminisced with me about his early days in peanut farming and some of the hard lessons he had learned about human nature. I learned a lot that day, more about human beings than about farm sales, and it was certainly worth more than the price of admission. Many of the men there bid on some items. But some were there because it was an event where they would be among people, pick up information, and while I doubt they would have called it this, prevent social isolation.

—Teddy

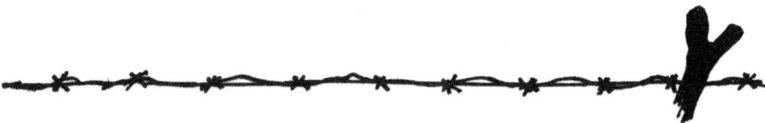

Capsule 94

The Story of Clarajane And The Red Hat Society

Clarajane Porter Dyess needed something to do. Her children were grown and gone, taking her grandchildren with them. Yes, they were still in Texas, but Texas is so big that when family moves to another part of the state, it can still be far away.

Her husband had his ranching activities to keep him busy, but Clarajane, or Cookie as she had been known since childhood, needed something. Something else besides the long-term care she was giving to her mother, a retired schoolteacher of 100 who now lived in an assisted facility some 30 miles from the ranch where she too had lived.

Cookie wasn't unhappy or bored or depressed, but she was in need of a social outlet. She found it in Spur, Texas, the largest town in Dickens County, with just over a thousand people.

Spur was 125 miles from the family ranch. Her husband Bob was a native Dickens County boy and still liked to go back home for class reunions and visits with old family friends. Cookie looked forward to these trips because it gave her the chance to socialize, too, for her husband's friends quickly had become her own.

Things in Spur, Texas, go slowly, too, and Cookie and the other women her age (which is never mentioned in polite Southern company) began to get the social urge at the same time. It's the kind of urge that propels you to take action, to unite, to join forces and say to the world,

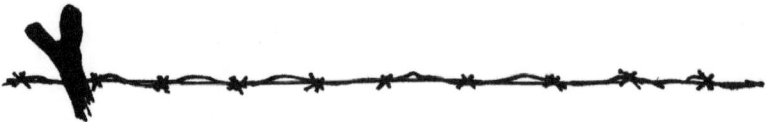

"Hey, we want a reason to get dressed up every now and then!" Thus began the N'Spurations, Dickens County's Red Hat Society.

It wasn't long before some 35–40 women joined this local chapter of the twentieth century analogy to the Crusades. Cookie, the only member of the N'Spurations living out of county, was given special exemption. The once-a-month meetings began to include teas and book reviews and luncheons, of course, and photo sessions. A southern social gathering of this magnitude must include photos, especially when the ladies were in full regalia of purple dresses and red hats.

Small towns are known for cliques, but what few women lived in Spur were equally welcome. The only requirement was to be over 60—that, after all, was what qualified you as "an old woman." Widowed ladies joined as did a 90-year old mother and her daughter.

The N'Spurations would borrow a church bus for some out-of-town tours to really big cities like Lubbock, 60 miles west of Spur on Highway 70. There they might make a visit to the mall or eat at some special restaurant since often this trip might be the only outing some of the truly elderly women would get to make each month.

Not all of their social gatherings were self-gratifying. At Christmas, the Red Hat Society of Spur decorated the nursing home, showing up in, of course, full regalia. The residents loved the colors and the attention that these N-spiring women offered. Photo sessions were especially moving in these settings as elderly and elderly posed for the cameras.

As with any social club, there was the occasional competitive element. When women dress up, they like to dress as no one else. They like to look better than their best and to outdo everyone else's best. The N'Spurations were no different. At one monthly meeting, Cookie became the unwilling instigator of a fashion trend as she appeared with a red lacy bra sewed and converted to a purse. It was so innovative and original that the other ladies had to have one. The next meeting many came with their own red bra purses. Then came the need to have bigger red bra

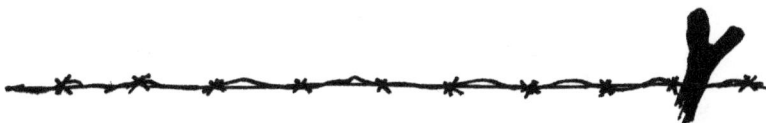

purses as the ladies tried to outdo their C-cup friends with double Ds. Finally, when it became apparent that size mattered to some, Cookie made an emotional plea to remember that the Red Hatters were not about bra sizes but about the size of their hearts. The tearful conclusion to the red bra purse episode culminated at the next year's homecoming bonfire when the N-Spurations met to burn their bras. They also had a great homecoming float, but for some reason the bra burning was more newsworthy in this small town.

Cookie still makes those 250 miles round trip excursions to Spur. She hasn't convinced anyone in Borden County to charter a Red Hat Society, but she isn't too disappointed. Borden County is for grandkids and ranching interests. Dickens County and the N'Spurations give Clarajane the underwire lift she needs.

—Sue Jane

Capsule 95

Tending To—It's What You Do

*P*eople whose life is close to the land are accustomed to tending. Tending means to minister to the needs of, to take care of. You tend to animals, the land, your family, the people in your community. It comes naturally, it seems, with the agricultural way of life. But some "tending to" comes more easily than others. For example, taking care of the details of the unpleasant possibilities of serious illness or death is a way of tending to our families, of making those situations easier for all concerned. But as kind and caring as it is to reduce the distress, we often put off having the discussions and making the decisions that will make those difficult times easier.

Each of us has probably known of a situation where a family must decide on behalf of a critically ill family member about the extent of treatment they should receive. "He's only 35. He has every reason to live," his mother says. The grandparent points out, "The doctor said he's in constant pain and the surgery has only a 20% chance of success." The young man's wife is too distraught to speak; she can only cry. Who makes the decision about cancer treatment for this unconscious patient? Another scene. Dad is 89. He's been confused and forgetful for the past three years since his wife died, has become progressively more demented and now has stopped eating. The children, ages 60 through 66, are

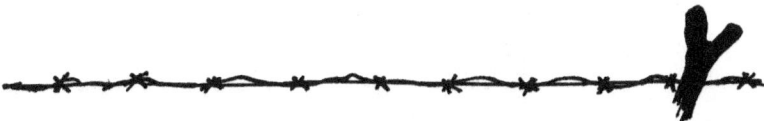

gathered in the nursing home to make a decision about inserting a feeding tube. Two say, "We can't let him starve." The other two say, "He's ready to go." The argument creates a major rift among the brothers and sisters.

Nothing makes these or similar situations pleasant or easy to endure. But, planning and developing Advance Directives can reduce the trauma. Although we may feel that this is primarily a concern for the aging, any one of us could be rendered unable to make decisions about our health care at any time as a result of disease or accident.

Two types of decisions can be made to provide direction for your care in case of your inability to make choices. One is called Durable Health Care Power of Attorney. The second is referred to as a Living Will. Together they are called Advance Medical Directives. The more comprehensive Advance Medical Directives document may also state preferences about organ donation, autopsy, and disposal of remains.

Deciding whom to designate to make health care decisions on your behalf is the most important choice to make. The person selected should understand the responsibility and you should be comfortable that they will make the type of decision you'd want to make if you were able. You'll have to communicate as you make the decision and at least each time you review your choice. This person becomes the health care decision maker only if you are unable but must know your wishes.

A Living Will is a document that states instructions about health care decisions that you wish to give, usually about end of life care including pain management and life-prolonging measures. There can be specific directions or simply guidelines to assist the decision maker.

An attorney can be an important resource to guide the process of developing the elements of Advance Directives. But, it's not a requirement that an attorney develop the documents. Several resources provide information and forms to create the documents. As state laws vary, it's important to use information specific to your state. Some good references are available at www.abanet.org/aging,

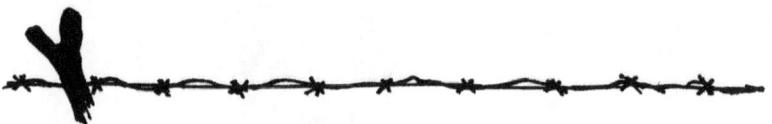

www.partnershipforcaring.org, and www.aarp.org (search for Advance Directives on this site).

When decisions about a person's health care must be made on their behalf, even the best written documents are a poor substitute for personal communication prior to the situation. Continuing communication is also important. A person's wishes may change during their life. The Advance Directives can be changed at any time to reflect this. No one wants to talk about the critical situations when Advance Directives would be used. But, talking about these issues and developing Advance Directives is one important way that folks who care can tend to their loved ones.

—Teddy

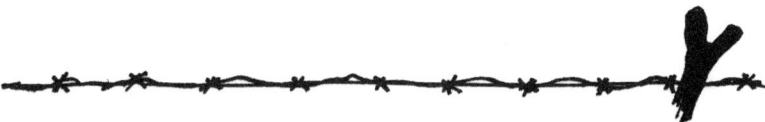

Capsule 96

Volunteer Voices

On Thomas Jefferson's grave marker, there is no mention of the fact that he was the third president of the United States.

At his insistence, the inscription mentions his authoring a rather famous declaration, overseeing the creation of the University of Virginia, and sponsoring a bill in his home state that would guarantee religious freedom. Those are the achievements for which he wanted to be remembered, not the fact that he held the highest political office in the land for eight years.

Jefferson regretted giving up his private life on his farm although he knew he needed to answer the call to serve. Within us all and more in some, exists a need to serve.

Often in rural areas, people crutch out of volunteering by noting that there are few organizations to join for such work. Since when does a person need an organization to visit the elderly in a community? Must we have library cards before we offer to read a book to the children down the road whose parents are out in the fields? Does the fact that there isn't a Kiwanis or Rotary Club in a community of 150 people mean that scholarships aren't to be made available for the graduating class of eight seniors?

Of all settings, the small town should have the desire to take care of its own. A volunteering spirit should be a natural extension of

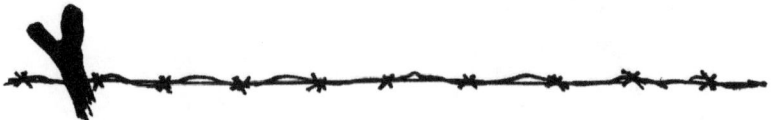

what is really a family atmosphere. Everyone does know everyone, and the more they reach out to help, the better the chances are that the community service will become contagious.

Perhaps this service might influence outsiders to move in to the community, helping preserve its very existence. School systems in particular have the power to boost a small town's population by being goodwill ambassadors as students and teachers alike participate in activities in outlying cities.

Organizations, however, are valid and ever present in even some small towns. One ladies Bible class visits a local nursing home twice a week to volunteer washing and rolling the residents' hair. Another town may not have an assisted living facility but does have a library. Groups such as Friends of the Library can be organized to support the local library with fundraisers. Budget cuts can jeopardize the ability of the library to purchase new books or provide educational services to the community, so raising money and awareness is crucial. A school's parents' club hosts an annual Fall Festival with booths and bake sales to fund scholarships for graduating seniors.

We need not use the excuse that "there's nothing to do" on a volunteer basis even if we live rurally. Thomas Jefferson's volunteer efforts created a new nation, a new university, and a new way of thinking.

The nearest gas station may be 35 miles away, but walking down a country road with the intent of lending a helping hand creates its own energy. Volunteering can go a long way towards replenishing rural communities.

—Sue Jane

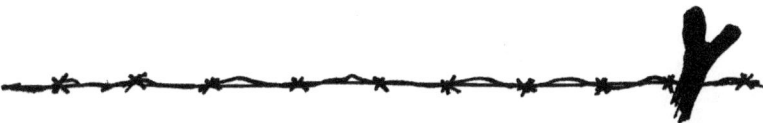

Capsule 97

On Reading The Last Paragraph First

The headline in the Bulletin of the AARP (American Association of Retired Persons) read "Self Exams Don't Reduce Breast Cancer Deaths." Because I've spent a lot of hours teaching women of all ages how to examine their breasts and reminding them to do so regularly, it caught my eye. I recalled that I had heard a similar bit of information on radio recently. The article was brief and the radio piece was only a sentence or two. Both the headline and the "sound bite" fit in the "Man Bites Dog" category. You know, it's not news when a dog bites a man. That's what dogs do. But when a man bites a dog, *that's news.*

I am convinced that a lot of what passes for health-related news these days is of the latter category. Even if the research on which the story is based, when read in full, gives a somewhat different picture, the headline is designed to catch the eye. A single controversial element is highlighted to attract the reader.

It worked. I read the headline—that one that was waving at me and all other card-carrying members of the AARP—and went on to the first paragraph. If I had stopped there, I would have abandoned my own breast self-exams and saved a lot of time trying to teach and encourage patients to do theirs. That first paragraph said, "...self-exams don't save lives." Whoa! What evidence is there, I wondered, to support this advice? (As you know, that's the same question any successful farmer or rancher

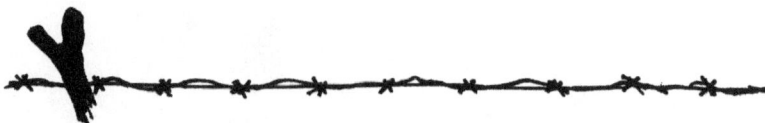

asks before radically changing an aspect of their operation.)

The article mentioned the name of the researcher. Checking out the research report "behind the headline," I gained some important facts.

For example, the research was performed in China, using a large sample (266,000 women) of factory workers. They were randomly placed in two groups. One group received special breast self-exam instruction and reminders. The other half of the women received no special instruction or reminders. After 10 years, the rate of death from breast cancer was approximately the same in both groups. That's where the headline writer grabbed a fact and ran. MAN BITES DOG!

Good scientists are careful to mention the limitations of their research. Even though the number of women in the study was large (a good feature of the design), this was a single study in one culture. No conscientious researcher makes generalizations about *all women* based on one study of women in China. To have confidence in the results, repeated studies must show the same results. And the head of this study, Dr. David B. Thomas, did what a good scientist should. He reported that, "...the results do not mean that women should stop self-exams but the self checks are no substitute for routine mammograms." There it was, in the last paragraph of the AARP article.

The headline writer had done his or her job-caught my eye. So, what's my point in all of this? There are two. First, do continue to do regular self-breast exams and follow your health care provider's recommendations for screening mammograms or diagnostic sonograms or other tests if problems are identified. If doing the self exams does nothing more than make a person familiar with changes in her body, that heightened awareness may encourage her to have the annual clinical exam and

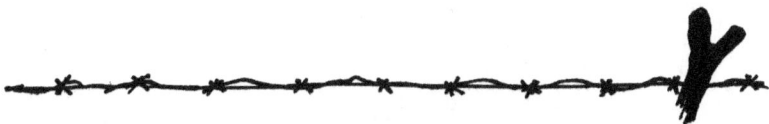

mammogram that are basic to diagnosing (and successfully treating) breast cancer. That awareness and prompting to have clinical exams and mammograms is certainly not as widespread as is needed to reduce deaths from breast cancer. What makes me say that? The American Cancer Society's data show that only about 50% of the women over 40 years of age in several of the farming and ranching states have had a clinical exam and mammogram in the past year.

Second, spread the word in your community that it's important to read (or listen to) all health-related news critically. The *bottom line* is often in the last paragraph.

—Teddy

Capsule 98

The Older The Better

*A*ging is inevitable, or at least we hope it is. The alternative to getting older is to die young. Most people aren't in favor of that. It's a pity then that we don't value the process of aging as well as honor the aged.

We could learn a great deal from the Hispanic culture where older men and women are referred to with new titles. Señor becomes "don" and señora "dona." With adulation and great respect, the Spanish culture places its elderly in a revered state.

Within our small communities, opportunity for interaction between older adults and school-age children should be created as often as possible. At a small local church, the few members attending may be either really young or really old. The children could learn important lessons of respect while the older adults can impart their wisdom. Some small congregations have begun Secret Grandparent programs. Children whose grandparents live far away can adopt grandparents within the community. Without identifying themselves, the children send cards or supply secret treats for their "grandparents" and a revealing party is held at the end of the school year.

The elderly in small rural communities have a responsibility, too, to continue their involvement in town or school activities. Self-pity is an easy trap for the aged. Some don't or can't drive, and staying home

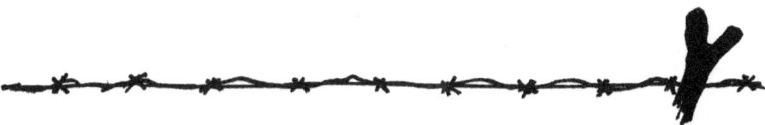

becomes a way of life. In small towns, however, distances to the school for a home ballgame shouldn't be deterrents. There's always a local teenager wanting to practice driving, so if someone needs a ride, the student council could set up a special taxi service for getting older people to functions like one-act plays, basketball or football games, church activities, or even to drink coffee down at the lone local café.

Little towns should never be guilty of letting anyone, much less the aged, get lost in the crowd. There is an almost automatic accessibility just because of the small population. The lesson for the younger generations is to develop an appreciation of and show a healthy respect for their elders. As for those in the senior citizen category, take a chance and get to know those kids. They might even like to drink a Coke and play a game of 42 in the backroom of the local gin.

Alfred Lord Tennyson gave these words to the epic hero Ulysses who, in preparing for one final journey as a weathered soldier, knew that he still had what it took to participate fully in life despite his old age:

> Come, my friends,
> 'Tis not too late to seek a newer world.
> Tho' much is taken, much abides, and tho'
> We are not now that strength
> Which in old days
> Moved earth and heaven,
> That which we are,
> We are—
> One equal temper of heroic hearts,
> Made weak by time and fate,
> But strong in will
> To strive, to seek, to find, and not to yield.

—Sue Jane

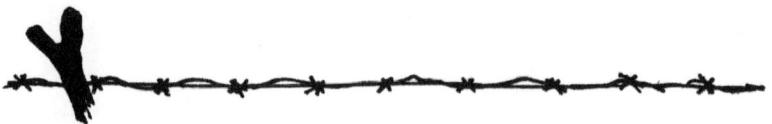

294

Capsule 99

Let Them Play

*T*yler was the Marshall Matt Dillon of our neighborhood. From his toddler days, he dressed as a cowboy, talked like a cowboy, walked like a cowboy. He even learned to play the guitar and sing just in case he was called on to perform around the neighborhood "campfire."

He did this until he was 12 years old. He probably would have continued to live this way had jr. high athletics not interrupted his lifestyle. Being forced to wear shorts in P.E. instead of jeans really burned his britches so to speak, but he loved football and made the concession.

In our small town, Tyler and my daughters and many other children who lived on the block were able to stretch their childhood years. They played outside, in the streets, on the practice football field in their backyards, or in the vacant lots overgrown with mesquite trees. Both boys and girls practiced roping and riding in anticipation of success in rodeo or on the ranch. They knew what snake holes to watch for, and they remembered to check in mid-morning and lunch to let some parental figure know where they were and whom they were with.

It was a utopian setting reminiscent of an earlier time in larger towns where children everywhere could be children for as long as they wanted. My own childhood in a town much larger than Gail allowed me the same freedoms as Tyler and his playmates. We could walk to

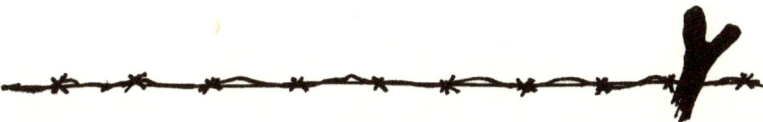

school and walk home for lunch and not have to sign out or be signed out by a certain person. It was the best of times.

Tyler is soon to graduate from high school in the same little town where he's grown up. He's tossed the cowboy gear but has kept his guitar. Preferring the Beatles and grunge bands like Nirvana, Tyler wears his jeans baggy, and they aren't Wranglers anymore.

I see him and the younger kids on the block today and see the cycle thankfully repeating itself. There are new cowboys and cowgirls playing on the dirt mounds around the school. As always, bicycle and scooter traffic keep me vigilant as I drive by and wave at the pleasant sight of children at play.

I wish I could convey to them just how lucky they are to have this small town in which to thrive. Would I tell them about the children in Sierra Leone who have been forced to fight in a war, killing other children as well as adults? Do these young neighbors of mine know about their Jewish and Palestinian counterparts who can't walk, much less play, safely down a street? And even in their own United States, do they know that children in cities face daily threats of drug dealers hoping to rein in a new innocent customer?

My maternal nature is torn between telling them about reality and protecting them from it. More than anything, I want to preserve and appreciate the status quo of my rural neighborhood.

However, there's no need to be naïve. Of course my little neighbors are not completely safe. Nor was I in my small town where a neighborhood boy molested me on more than one occasion.

But I can't help but be thankful that I still see lemonade stands across the street and forts built out of cardboard boxes. The kid with the slip and slide is still the coolest, and the guy who lives on a ranch and gets to shoot his BB gun in the pasture is envied. Walking to the store for an afternoon soft drink and candy bar is an after-school routine.

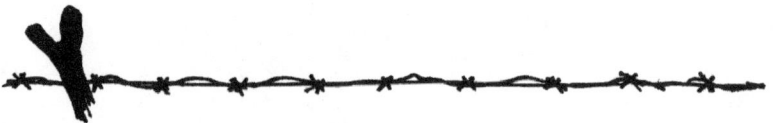

Safe and sound.

Thankfully the norm in small communities, but what children everywhere deserve.

—Sue Jane

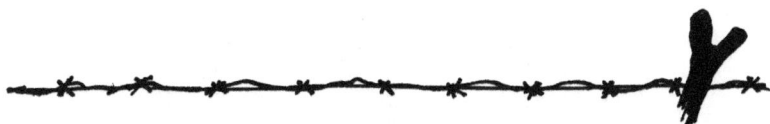

Capsule 100

A Dose of Reality

My English II class was all abuzz recently about one of those reality television shows. Oh, that they could get that excited over Shakespeare.

I try to tell them that Romeo and Juliet's situation is much more realistic. Kids fall in love, their parents disapprove, they react, etc. You tell me when the last time was that seven good-looking bachelors made fools of themselves over any of us? How about reality shows about plastic surgery? Maybe I could refer to those to teach irony.

Reality television is hardly the real thing.

Unfortunately, that's the way many elements of society are today. The so-called reality of economics is that many people work less and make more money. Actually, the reverse is true, that many people work more and make less. In the field of medicine, the reality is that you pay more for health care and get less attention due to a *real* shortage in the nursing field.

Political "realities" depend on election year dynamics or personal agendas. Very few historical examples exist of intervention in Africa to help with real problems those people have faced for generations.

Most people wouldn't recognize reality if it walked up to them and slapped them in the face.

This book has included doses of healthy advice, humorous

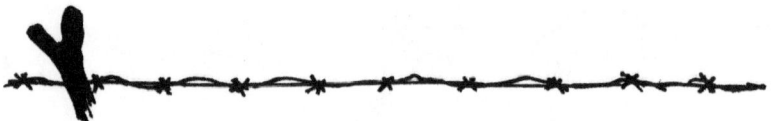

reflections, and practical life lessons. All contain a dose of reality. Real things make us smile, make us laugh out loud, make us sad, make us weep, and usually make us think. Above all, real things should make us better people.

In Margery Williams children's classic, *The Velveteen Rabbit*, the stuffed animals in a child's nursery are discussing what makes something real. In the exchange below, the old Skin Horse shares with the new Rabbit how reality happens.

"The Skin Horse had lived longer in the nursery than any of the others. He was so old that his brown coat was bald in patches and showed the seams underneath, and most of the hairs in his tail had been pulled out to string bead necklaces. He was wise, for he had seen a long succession of mechanical toys arrive to boast and swagger, and by-and-by break their mainsprings and pass away, and he knew that they were only toys, and would never turn into anything else. For nursery magic is very strange and wonderful, and only those playthings that are old and wise and experienced like the Skin Horse understand all about it.

'What is real?" asked the Rabbit one day, when they were lying side by side near the nursery fender, before Nana came to tidy the room. 'Does it mean having things that buzz inside you and a stick-out handle?'

'Real isn't how you are made," said the Skin Horse. 'It's a thing that happens to you. When a child loves you for a long, long time, not just to play with, but really loves you, then you become Real.'

'Does it hurt?' asked the Rabbit.

'Sometimes,' said the Skin Horse, for he was always truthful. 'When you are Real you don't mind being hurt.'

'Does it happen all at once, like being wound up,' he asked, 'or bit by bit?'

'It doesn't happen all at once,' said the Skin Horse. 'You become. It takes a long time. That's why it doesn't happen often to people who break easily, or have sharp edges, or who have to be carefully kept.

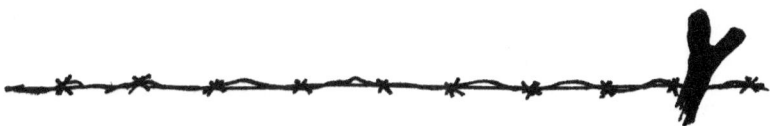

Generally, by the time you are Real, most of your hair has been loved off, and your eyes drop out and you get loose in your joints and very shabby. But these things don't matter at all, because once you are Real you can't be ugly, except to people who don't understand.'"

My students probably wouldn't like to read the rest of this story because it isn't about real people. A story about stuffed animals would come across as childish to a teenager and to some adults.

At some point we must all realize that real things are rooted in those relationships and situations where we learn more about ourselves. I never met my grandmother, but listening to stories about her and then writing about them has taught me many lessons. That's reality.

During my teenage years, I never wanted to talk to my mother. Now, I can't seem to get enough of her. Recording her childhood memories in this book has heightened my awareness of her strength. That's reality.

Somehow, I don't think I'll ever find myself trying to survive in a jungle or walking across a skyscraper blindfolded just to out-fear someone.

It won't be long before I will want to tell my grandchildren stories about their great-great grandmother's evening walks across the pastures on the Fisher County farm. Then I'll tell them about their great-grandmother's Saturday Shirley Temple matinees in little Rotan, Texas. Finally, a story or two about my brothers and sisters' backyard forts, sandlot baseball games, and horned toad hunts should either make them giggle or put them to sleep.

Not quite television programming material, but these stories will be commercial free and very, very real.

—Sue Jane

 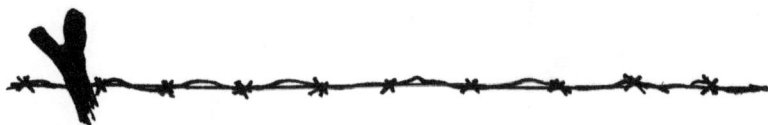